CONTENTS

ABOUT THE AUTHORS:

Dr Chloë-Maryse Baxter BSc(Hons) MB ChB with European Studies (Manchester)

Chloë Baxter graduated from Manchester Medical School in 2001, MB ChB with European Studies, having also obtained an intercalated BSc in Health Care Ethics and Law. At the time of writing she was a Pre-Registration House Officer in Edinburgh. She is currently a Senior House Officer in Sydney, Australia, studying part-time for the Masters in Health Professions Education at Maastricht University in the Netherlands.

Mark G Brennan BA(Hons) (Surrey) MA (London) AKC DHMSA ILTM FRIPH

Mark Brennan obtained his MA in Medical Law and Ethics at Kings College London in 1991, and is a Lecturer in Medical & Dental Education at the University of Wales College of Medicine in Cardiff. He is Visiting Senior Lecturer in Medical Ethics at the Royal College of Surgeons in Ireland; Visiting Senior Lecturer at Trinity College Dublin; and Honorary Research Fellow at the Centre for Ethics in Medicine at the University of Bristol.

Dr Yvette G M Coldicott BSc(Hons) MB ChB (Bristol)

Yvette Coldicott was a final year medical student at Bristol University when the book was written; she also obtained an intercalated BSc in Bioethics. She is now a Pre-Registration House Officer at Bristol Royal Infirmary (UBHT). She teaches medical ethics and law to students and doctors.

Acknowledgements

We dedicate this book to our families and friends; those who taught each of us about medical ethics in practice, and those whom we now teach; our patients and colleagues in healthcare; our team of international contributors; with thanks for all their support, encouragement and inspiration.

CONTRIBUTORS

Dr Shrilla Banerjee, London, England
Dr Jamiu Busari, Netherlands Antilles
Dr Alejandro Cragno, Buenos Aires, Argentina
Dr Stephen Child, Auckland, New Zealand
Dr Sophie Frankland, London, England
Prof Michel Gillet, Lausanne, Switzerland
Dr Nermin Halkic, Lausanne, Switzerland
Dr Richard Huxtable, Bristol, England
Associate Prof Mitchell Levy, Providence (RI), USA
Dr Vassilis Lykomitros, Athens, Greece
Dr Dhruv Mankad, Nasik, India
Prof Marcellina Mian, Toronto, Canada
Ms Maaike Möller, The Netherlands
Dr Elizabeth Morris, Edinburgh, Scotland
Dr Peter Mills, London, England
Dr Emma Nelson, Dublin, Ireland
Dr Jonathan Osborn, Bristol, England
Prof Graham Ramsay, Maastrict, The Netherlands
Prof Peter Rosen, San Diego (CA), USA
Dr Francesca Rubulotta, Providence (RI), USA
Dr Joan Saary, Toronto, Canada
Dr Emma Sedgwick, London, England
Dr Adrian Sutton, Manchester, England
Dr Andy Swain, Palmerston North, New Zealand
Dr Bob Taylor, Belfast, Northern Ireland
Dr Anthony Toft, Edinburgh, Scotland
Dr Hamish Wallace, Edinburgh, Scotland
Associate Prof Merilynn Walton, Sydney, Australia

PERMISSIONS

PasTest would like to thank the following for allowing material to be used in this book:

British Medical Association
Eating Disorders Association
General Medical Council

FOREWORD

Associate Professor Jill Gordon

Head of Medical Education Unit and Associate Dean, Faculty of Medicine, University of Sydney, Australia

MB BS (University of Sydney), BA (University of Newcastle), MPsychMed (University of New South Wales), PhD (University of Newcastle), FRACGP.

In 1908, John Dewey and James Tufts wrote:

> "the (moral) theorist ... must take his departure from the problems which men actually meet in their own conduct. He may define and refine these; he may divide and systematise; he may abstract the problems from their concrete contexts in individual lives... but if he gets away from them, he is talking about something his own brain has invented, not about moral realities."

This book deals with 'moral realities' that will stimulate reflection for doctors at every level. You won't find these ethical dilemmas on the front page of the newspaper or in the evening news on TV, but they are of the kinds that affect more lives than most of the exotic issues found in the headlines. Rather than portraying doctors as white knights or black demons, they capture the complexities of life as a junior doctor or medical student.

The problem inherent in any dilemma can be found in the definition of the word itself. A dilemma is concerned with two valid but opposed propositions. Assuming that neither proposition can be invalidated, a dilemma can never be fully resolved. The problem of competing rights, such as those that apply to pregnant women and their unborn babies, is a classic example.

Day to day practice is full of simple but important dilemmas – whether or not to provide a patient with certain information, to recommend a test or use a particular treatment. Even in the course of making 'ordinary' clinical decisions, thoughtful doctors know that they might have made another choice. We cannot know where that other decision may have led us and our patients, and we cannot be certain of having done the greatest good and the least possible harm in every case, no matter how hard we try. Lawyers operate with the benefit of retrospect to cope, but doctors cope with the untidiness of the 'here and now'.

Doctors can be tempted to seek a greater sense of certainty. They can:

- fail to notice that ethical dilemmas exist;
- treat each dilemma as if it were simply a debate which can be won or lost; or
- behave as though ethical dilemmas can be resolved by technical means – that given 'enough science' the right answer will eventually reveal itself.

The real life examples in this book illustrate why it is that these responses are bound to be unsatisfactory. Doctors who fail to notice the presence of a multitude of ethical dilemmas also fail to grow, both personally and professionally. Doctors who think dilemmas can be 'won or lost' like debates deny the subtlety and complexity of their human experience. The reductionists reduce not only the ethical challenge, but themselves.

By contrast, the contributors to this book show that they know just how uncertain medicine can be. Medical students and junior doctors who wonder if they are the only people who have not yet found the One Right Answer can rest assured that dilemmas are just that – unresolved questions that nevertheless demand practical responses.

Paradoxically, the experiences described in this book do not justify a position of ethical nihilism. They demonstrate, among other things, the importance of virtue as a guide to action. William Osler was drawn to the conclusion that:

> "the greatest therapeutic gifts are kindness, human understanding, sympathy and common sense (which) in a continually changing scientific world ... remain permanently desirable attributes."

Congratulations to Chloë Baxter, Mark Brennan and Yvette Coldicott for gathering these stories together. They have enriched the contributions with their own valuable experiences, both medical and ethical, to create a 'therapeutic gift' to their readership.

CHAPTER 1:
INTRODUCTION

Welcome to the practical guide to medical ethics and law! While the book is intended for junior doctors and medical students, we hope it will also be of interest to teachers of medical ethics and law, and to other medical teachers, health professionals and medical scientists.

The main body of the book is made up of case studies. Studying clinical cases is the most efficient way to learn anything in medicine, and ethics and law is no exception.

You will find two types of cases in the book.

The first cases have been worked out for you, giving a clear structure for approaching ethical and legal problems. All of these cases are based on real life situations which are known to the authors, or which have been described to us by our friends and colleagues. Mostly, they are a composite of incidents and events involving a range of patients, medical students and doctors in both hospital and primary care settings. Patients' and doctors' details have both been altered in order to ensure anonymity and protect confidentiality.

You can use these cases in three different ways:

- You can work through them on your own in stages, noting down your thoughts as you go.
- You can work through them with others in a group. This is the most efficient way in which to cover the issues since you can discuss and debate various points of view together. Working in a group is obviously good practice for working life as a doctor, because it requires you to tolerate and accept the existence of alternative views, and yet justify and defend your arguments to yourself and others. It is also good practice for exams.
- You can read through them as a revision exercise. Key revision points are indicated so you can easily spot them, and each case is summarised.

The second type (Chapter 5) are cases which come from doctors from all over the world. They are real life examples of ethico-legal dilemmas in clinical practice, and illustrate that even the most experienced clinicians find ethical dilemmas difficult to deal with. Patient details have been altered to maintain confidentiality.

SO WHY STUDY MEDICAL ETHICS AND LAW?

A young Bristol vet said recently: *"Your patients won't care how much you know, but they will know how much you care"*.

He was talking about caring for animals but he might just as well have been talking about people. Part of caring for people as a doctor is behaving in a way which is both ethically and legally acceptable. You could be the most knowledgeable doctor in the world, or the most technically competent in a given area, but without an ethical base to your medical practice, how good a doctor will you really be?

It wasn't long ago that the sum total of ethics teaching for the average British medical graduate consisted of a one-hour lecture by the Dean. In this, students were exhorted to obey the following commandments:

- not to advertise their services;
- not to get drunk on duty; and
- not to seduce their married patients.

These were popularly known as The Three A's (Advertising, Alcohol, and Adultery). There was little – if any – opportunity for formal discussion of ethical problems in medicine, as a student. Rather, it was assumed that the new medical graduate would be able to cope, surrounded as he or she was by what Professor Len Doyal has described as "well-disposed physicians". Of course these discussions still occurred informally, in the bar, in the mess, and in the library, but often without any authoritative teaching to assist the students in dealing with their inevitable concerns.

We firmly believe most people who choose to study and practise medicine do so with the best of intentions and motivations. They want to be – and be seen as – good doctors. We asked a group of junior doctors how they defined the qualities of a 'good' doctor. They came up with the following:

- A good communicator
- Clinically competent
- An improver of other people's health, and facilitator of access to healthcare
- Teacher – of patients, families, other doctors, medical students and health professionals
- Good listener and able to explain clearly
- Empathetic and sympathetic
- Patient and tolerant; non-discriminatory
- Genuine and kind
- Non-judgemental
- Fair and trustworthy

This list is not comprehensive or exclusive, nor does it mean that you will display all of these qualities on any one given day. Contrary to the expectations of some, doctors and medical students are human beings too, so they are fallible, imperfect, and likely to under-perform or even fail on occasions. Sometimes the pressures of working in medicine and in the health service can affect one's ability to be as good a doctor as one would want to be or should be. Patients can be amazingly forgiving and tolerant when doctors make mistakes, **if** that doctor displays some humility, says sorry where appropriate, appears caring, and keeps the patient informed of what is happening.

However, the above list **is** aspirational. It shows that, despite all the pressures and the all-too-frequent criticism of the medical profession, the majority of doctors regard what they do as more than just a job, and – now and then – recognise what a huge privilege it is to be part of one of the most respected professions.

Most doctors are conscientious individuals who reflect on the way they practise, occasionally to the point of obsession; they are concerned about getting it right.

Ethics (like the practice of medicine) is rarely about black and white, but about learning to discern the shades of grey, deal with uncertainty, and find the best possible course of action under the circumstances. We hope that this book will help you to think through possible courses of action or inaction in relation to the cases we present, the majority of which are drawn from personal experience and real life.

This book will not just help you prepare for your examinations and coursework, but will also remove some of the anxiety when you are a house officer, senior house officer, hospital or general practice registrar confronted with an ethical dilemma at 3 o'clock in the morning.

While this book is aimed primarily at doctors and medical students in the UK, we hope that the range of cases presented from around the world will make it useful to a wider audience. However, throughout the text, references will be made to the UK legal system and to the National Health Service.

CHAPTER 2:
HOW TO STUDY
ETHICS AND LAW

The first thing to say about studying medical ethics and law is start with an open mind.

As a medical student and doctor you have to know about relevant ethico-legal aspects at all levels of your career. Formal assessment of knowledge of ethics and law is becoming increasingly important as the Government and General Medical Council are requiring doctors and medical students to know what is expected of them; ignorance is not a defence. Medical schools and Royal Colleges are therefore examining ethics and law more overtly.

HOW TO REVISE FOR AND PASS THE EXAMS

What are OSCEs and what do they do?

Objective Structured Clinical Examinations (OSCEs) are now being used widely to examine students. They are primarily used to help assess clinical and communication skills as well as attitudes; they are also used to assess knowledge about ethical and legal issues.

OSCE formats

The format for these exams varies. An OSCE is usually made up of several 'stations', with each station lasting between five to ten minutes. A station is often a structured viva with certain props such as radiographs, blood results, or anatomical models. Real or standardised patients are frequently used too, especially to assess communication and examination skills. At least one examiner is present, to watch how you perform, ask you questions, or play a specific role, e.g. as a patient.

Marking

Marking schemes vary. Examiners will assess you by using either a checklist of items, a global rating scale, or a mixture of both.

- **Checklists** mean that you will only get credit for doing the things on the checklist. Your final mark for the station will be a reflection of how many items you managed to do successfully. However, checklists do not allow you to gain more marks for doing extra things not included on the checklist.
- **Global rating scales** mean that the examiner will look at your whole performance and give you the mark that is most appropriate. A marking guide is often followed so that examiners are aware of what standards of

performance equate to which mark. They allow examiners to give credit to a student who achieves everything required in a courteous, confident manner whereas a checklist may dictate that such a candidate receives the same mark as a student who does everything in a hesitant and disrespectful way.

Most examining bodies employ a mixture of both assessment formats. Examiners use a checklist to help them assess performance but ultimately they are asked to write down the mark they feel most appropriate based on overall competence.

Passing

Generally speaking, in order to do very well in an OSCE you will have to do well in most stations and in order to fail you have to perform poorly in most stations – most people pass.

There are three main ways used by examining bodies to decide who passes and who fails.

- **Criterion-referenced grading** means that candidates are assessed against a set of criteria and must reach a minimum standard or percentage (the 'passmark') in order to pass. This percentage is usually set before the exam takes place. Criterion-referencing means that as long as you achieve the predetermined percentage you will pass, no matter how many other candidates achieve the standard. However, if the exam is harder or easier than usual, it becomes unfair as fewer or more students respectively will manage to pass.
- **Norm-referenced grading** means that students are judged against each other. After the exam, all the marks are placed on a graph. A normal distribution curve (a bell-shaped line) inevitably results due to the fact that there are a small number of students who do very well and a small number who do poorly, with the majority achieving somewhere in between. Statistics using these results allow examining bodies to set a pass mark based on the performance of the students, so that the standard of the exam itself is less important. Norm-referencing is sometimes preferred because it is difficult to ensure that exactly the same standard of exam can be reproduced year after year. It is also good because you are compared against your peers, not against an arbitrary percentage. However, it also means that some students will inevitably fail each time, independent of their final percentage. Royal Colleges use this type of grading to decide which candidates pass and which fail their Membership exams.

- **Pass/Fail criteria.** Some stations have a pass/fail criterion which means that if you fail to do something then you will automatically fail the station no matter how well you perform overall. The pass/fail criterion is often something either very basic or very important, and usually it is both e.g. failing to check that other people are standing clear of the patient before defibrillating during advanced life support. It is also possible that an OSCE will have a pass/fail station which means that if you fail the station then you will automatically fail the entire OSCE no matter what your total score. Again, this station is likely to be examining something like basic life support – a fundamental skill. Most medical schools do not use pass/fail criteria and do not have pass/fail stations.

Ethics and law in OSCEs

There are several ways in which ethics and law can be brought into OSCEs.

A **whole** station may be purely about ethico-legal issues. You will be required to discuss ethico-legal principles for 5–10 minutes with an examiner or do a role play in that time. Real life examples that the authors have encountered are:

- Mental Health Act – when and why it may be necessary to section someone and how you should go about it
- Consent – talking to the mother of a child with an undescended testis; criteria for informed consent for treatment.
- Good medical practice – talking about what you would do if one of your colleagues was on drugs/alcohol and potentially unsafe to practise
- Refusal of consent to an operation – how to deal with this ethically and legally
- Child abuse/bullying – what to do if you suspect child abuse/bullying is happening, including issues surrounding breaching confidentiality
- Treatment in the best interests of the patient – how to deal with an unconscious patient who has attempted suicide

Ethico-legal issues can form **part** of a station. You may be required to draw upon and demonstrate ethico-legal knowledge in stations that primarily are designed to test other skills or knowledge. This occurs in many different scenarios and we have come across it in stations concerning:

- Taking a history of child abuse
- Discussing a positive result for a sexually transmitted infection with a patient
- Doing a cervical smear + colposcopy exam
- Discussing breastfeeding with a new mother – respecting her right to choose

- Management of a patient who has taken a paracetamol overdose
- Doing any kind of clinical exam, e.g. thyroid, rectal, chest – obtaining consent

Your situation

In order to prepare for an OSCE it is helpful to think about your own situation.

- What kind of skills and knowledge does your medical school usually examine?
- What stations have they done in the past?
- What are the obvious ethico-legal areas that are normally examined as entire stations?
- Are there any other stations that might involve ethico-legal aspects even though they might be primarily assessing other skills/knowledge?

Ten top tips for OSCEs

Before the OSCE:

1 Practise the skills in preparation for the OSCE.

Practice (with feedback) is the best way to improve any skill. In terms of ethico-legal skills this means confronting yourself with ethical and legal problems and thinking about how you would deal with them. The cases in this book are ideal to help you prepare. Work in groups so that you can give feedback to each other. Answer the questions above so you can tailor your revision to your own situation.

2 Get a good night's sleep before the exam.

OSCEs are usually about how you perform skills, not reproducing isolated facts. While you may feel that it is sometimes better to stay up late revising for an MCQ (which tests purely knowledge), an OSCE is a test that requires you to be fully mentally alert. You will not make a good impression if you look tired, unshaven or are scruffily dressed. Be well rested and confident.

During the OSCE:

3 Be prepared for ethico-legal issues to come up.

Do not be blinkered into seeing only clinical knowledge and skills as being relevant. Be aware that, just like everyday clinical practice, ethics and law pervades most aspects of medical care and therefore may come up in nearly any OSCE station.

4   Cite the issues that make the problem ethically or legally difficult.

When faced with an ethical dilemma such as the poorly performing colleague who may be endangering patient care, take a while to think about the issues before opening your mouth. For example, the fact that the colleague is a doctor and has a duty to their patients, the fact that you are a doctor and have a similar duty to patients, that telling on your colleague may not necessarily achieve the best outcome. Take your time to think about the problem from all angles. Show the examiner that you are exploring all the issues without rushing into action. Doing this will also give you time to think.

5   Take your time to go through the steps in your thought process.

Do not come up with solutions straight away. Examiners want to see that you are a careful decision-maker and that you will take time to examine the issues before making a judgement. They want you to demonstrate that you will think through such difficult problems in a clear and step-wise fashion. This shows that you are not simply a robot who has learned the 'answers' to several different ethical dilemmas, but that you are a thinking person who will address each situation on a case by case basis.

6   Know about the GMC 'Duties of a Doctor' guidance

These handbooks should be read before the exam so you can refer to them during the OSCE. You don't have to know page numbers or anything, but you should at least be aware that they exist and that they provide guidance on your responsibilities as a doctor. Mention it in the exam if it is relevant to do so.

7   Back up your thoughts by referring to ethical principles and approaches; show awareness of legal terms.

Refer by name to any ethical principles that you use, e.g. beneficence, utilitarianism. Explain any legal background to terms such as 'negligence' or 'capacity to give informed consent' if relevant. This tip will earn you brownie points only if you know what you are talking about! Do not use words if you are not sure what they mean – examiners will pick up on this and quiz you until you feel like you don't know anything at all. Stick to what you know, but if you know any ethical principles or legal terms so much the better.

8   Seek help.

The complicated nature of ethico-legal problems means that you would be unwise to act alone. Always say that you would seek help from a suitable source, e.g. a defence organisation, a senior, etc. Bear in mind safeguarding confidentiality when saying that you would do this.

9   Start each station with a positive attitude.

If you feel that you have done badly in a station forget about it as soon as the bell goes. Put it out of your mind and go into the next station with a clear head, fresh start and confident approach. Remember that in order to do badly in an OSCE you would have to do poorly in **most** stations. Even students who gain top marks tend to have at least one station that did not go well.

After the OSCE:

10   Relax with your mates.

The OSCE is often a very stressful experience since it usually requires you to demonstrate a diverse range of skills under time pressure. It is important to relax and unwind afterwards in whatever way you please. Dissect the exam with your friends if you must, but remember that the OSCE is a very individual experience and it is almost impossible to know how your performance compares to anyone else's. Wait until the results come out before you cancel your summer holiday!

Ethics and law in essays

Most of us will not have had much practice at essay writing, especially now that medical schools are moving away from using essays to assess knowledge. Despite this, it is still a useful skill to learn and will help you in the future when you are asked to write papers, reports and book chapters.

Essay formats and marking

Writing essays in ethics and law can come in various formats. It could be as a special study module (SSM), a piece of coursework, or as a formal exam done under time pressure.

Essays can be marked in various ways. Sometimes examiners will use a checklist to ensure that you have covered the relevant points. You may also get credit for writing well; a clear structure and style, logical arguments and conclusions, spelling and referencing are all important.

Ten top tips for writing an essay

Before the essay:

1   Have a positive attitude.

OK, so you may not rate yourself as much of a writer but doing an essay is not that scary. You are intelligent, can think logically, and can cope with new challenges – that's all you need to start off with. You can do this.

2   Pick a topic that interests you.

Whether it is for an SSM or an exam, you will often be given several options from which to choose to write about. Think about issues that grab you and stimulate you in some way. It need not be something you know a lot about already, but if the topic inspires you to **think** in the first place then you will learn much more easily. In the early stages it is much better to be passionate about the subject than know a lot about it.

3   Increase your background knowledge of the subject.

Research the topic in the library. Use journals as well as books so that you learn about how different people have approached the topic. Compare your viewpoint with theirs: do they agree with you? In what respect do they disagree with you? What are the flaws in their arguments? All this can be included in your essay.

4   Discuss your thoughts with others.

Debating the issues with others will help you to detect holes in your arguments, and develop a wider perspective. The good thing about this is that you can start up discussions with anyone who's interested. Most people have opinions even if they can't back them up very well. Talk to other medics or other students, doctors, patients, your family and friends – this is what happens in real practice.

5   Make a plan.

This is the key to a good essay. If you have a good plan then your writing will flow much better. Note down the main aspects that you are going to address. A very basic plan may be along the lines of:

- Introduction – the context of the problem/case description
- Breakdown of the relevant ethical/legal issues
- Examination of each issue in turn – what your argument is, the opposing position, and why your position is stronger
- Summary of the final conclusion

Your plan should be more detailed than this, and you should be able to use the headings in your final essay. If possible, discuss your plan with your supervisor so that they can give you some feedback on your ideas and you can make sure you are on the right track. In an exam, make sure you put a line through your plan before handing it in.

During the essay:

6   Get yourself in the right mood and environment.

You'll need to get yourself into a quiet place with no distractions. Most people prefer to write on a computer but you must do what you're most comfortable with. If you prefer to handwrite your work then get lots of paper and a good pen.

7 Be disciplined and start writing.

The hardest thing about writing an essay is getting started. Do not make it into a psychological barrier that you have to break through. Just sit down and do it. You can always change the introduction later on if you're not happy with it. If necessary you can create rewards for yourself when you have achieved certain targets along the way. Chocolate is always a good one, but it could be anything that you enjoy. Make sure you take regular breaks too.

8 Don't worry:

- **about the word count** – you will find enough to write about; just make sure you don't waffle or repeat yourself;
- **if you get stuck** – take a break, go and do something else, talk to your supervisor;
- **about using simple language** – write in the best way you can to express what you think. It is always better to say complicated things in a simple way than simple things in a complicated way.

9 Check through the essay before handing it in.

Get other people to read it through too if possible, to get a fresh perspective on what you've written. Sometimes you can get so close to it that you fail to see obvious mistakes. If you have time, leave the essay alone for a few days and look at it again yourself. It should be easy to read, flow logically, be well structured with headings and have each argument backed up with references.

After the essay:

10 Get feedback.

You may want to forget about the essay once you've handed it in. However, use each assignment as an opportunity to get better. Try to get specific feedback from the examiner about areas you can improve for next time. Examples of common problems include lack of clarity in your explanation, illogical steps in your arguments, or being too waffly.

WHY I DID A BSC...

If you are thinking about studying medical ethics and law in greater depth there are several options open to you. You could decide to do a Special Study Module (SSM), an intercalated BSc or even a postgraduate degree.

Here are the personal thoughts of one of the authors (Chloë Baxter) on the experience of doing an intercalated BSc.

"I had several very clear reasons for doing a BSc in medical ethics and law.

Interest in the subject; desire to take a year out of science

The main reason was that I was interested in the subject. I think this is essential and would not recommend doing a BSc in **anything** unless you are interested in it. I realised that I had spent most of my time in formal education increasing my knowledge of science and developing a scientific approach to problems. This is undoubtedly useful but there is a lot more to medicine than science. I believe studying philosophy and ethics has helped me to think outside 'the box' and appreciate different aspects of human problems.

Wish to develop my own ethical beliefs and debating skills

One of the most inspiring teachers that I came into contact with during the pre-clinical years was the professor of medical ethics. He used to challenge over 200 students at a time to come up with answers to ethical problems. His lectures and debates were always very passionate and involving. I became motivated to learn more about my own beliefs and to discover why I thought the way I thought. During the BSc course itself I also learned debating skills and how to structure my arguments convincingly so that I could justify my position.

Wish to improve my essay writing technique

I reluctantly realised that being able to write essays is a useful skill and would help me to improve my written communication. However, I didn't like doing it and had strategically managed to avoid it since the age of 16 (choosing science subjects for A-levels). Medical ethics and law courses usually involve a lot of essay writing. I did find it very difficult at first but lecturers are used to dealing with students who have little essay writing experience and gave very good support. By the end of the course, I had more or less conquered my essay writing phobia and sometimes it was even enjoyable!

Getting an extra qualification

An intercalated degree is definitely a good bargain – you get a three year degree for the price of one. If you want to do a BSc because you'd like some extra letters after your name that is fair enough since it will be an advantage to your career. However, I would strongly advise you to pick a subject you enjoy. Spending a year forcing yourself to become immersed in something you dislike is a recipe for torture and failure. If you can't find anything you like at the moment then wait a year or two. There are always new courses starting up on different subjects in different places. Most medical schools allow you to intercalate at any time before your final year. Further possibilities will be open to you as you continue in your postgraduate career, e.g. Masters or PhD degrees. Medical ethics and law is also available as an MA or MSc so you could always pursue the interest after you have graduated from medicine instead of doing an intercalated BSc.

Spending an extra year as a student

This can be seen as a disadvantage by some people but for me it was definitely a plus point. There are of course some problems: you may become a year behind friends who continue on the medical course, your debt will increase, you may feel that you will forget some medical knowledge during your year 'out'. I experienced all of these problems but to a much smaller degree than I expected.

- Instead of losing friends, you gain them. It was also useful to have good mates in the year above who could tell me what to expect in exams and teach me on the wards.
- Money can be a worry and if it is an issue for you, there are trust funds around which may be able to help. Speak to your medical society, faculty, Student Union and bank about ways in which you can minimise the financial burden of extending your studies.
- Forgetting medical knowledge happens to some extent but you will be surprised by how much you retain. You will also be at an advantage compared to others in your year as you will know a lot of ethics and law which will be useful for your medical exams both at undergraduate and postgraduate level.

Being a student is ultimately very enjoyable and allows you to take some more long summer holidays – which you will miss greatly once you start work. Make the most of it!

As a Pre-Registration House Officer

Working as a PRHO in paediatrics, paediatric surgery and adult medicine I am constantly surprised by how much I have used my training in ethics and law. It sounds like a cliché, but every day I come across situations where I have to make ethical decisions or know relevant medical law. I can only see this knowledge becoming more essential as I progress further in my post-graduate career. The more senior and experienced you become, the more responsibility you will have and the more important and difficult the decisions you will be required to make.

Picking a course

If your university offers an intercalated degree option in medical ethics and law then the easiest thing to do is apply for that one. However, several places offer such a course so it may be worthwhile investigating the alternatives. Factors which you may want to take into account include:

- **Method of teaching**

Discussions and debates based on relevant problems are the best and usually the most enjoyable way in which to learn medical ethics and law. The course I did was run jointly with an MA in Health Care Ethics and Law and the people doing the MA were healthcare professionals themselves. This made for very lively and interesting discussions and most people had real life experience which they brought into group sessions. I found this motivating and learned a great deal more about practical applications of ethico-legal principles due to this particular virtue of the course.

- **Flexibility of the course to suit your interests**

Is the course modular? Which parts are compulsory and what are the options available to choose from?

- **Method of assessment**

Will you be assessed continuously or by an exam at the end? Maybe there is a mixture of both. It is likely that most courses use essay assignments to evaluate students but there may be other methods, e.g. MCQs, oral presentations, etc.

- **Students and teachers' views**

Speak to people who are on the course or who have completed it; arrange a meeting with one of the lecturers or course organisers.

What are the students' views? Did they enjoy the course? If they had difficulties, was there good support from the lecturers? Do the course organisers listen to suggestions on ways to improve the course and has action been taken in response to problems? Good and enthusiastic lecturers will be only too pleased to discuss the course with you. You will also create a good impression because you are making an effort to find out about the course in advance.

• Location

If you decide you want to go to a different university to do your BSc it is a good idea to familiarise yourself with the location. Investigate areas like accommodation, the student union, facilities, libraries, etc. Moving away for a year can be difficult initially but is often a fantastic experience."

CHAPTER 3:
THE BASICS OF
MEDICAL ETHICS
AND LAW

PHILOSOPHICAL

We have produced a doctor's 'rough guide' to help you understand the philosophical jargon, and the ideas behind the main theories. This glossary will be useful for exams, writing essays and when you are reading ethical texts.

Codes

Hippocratic Oath: The first ethical code of conduct for doctors. Composed by Hippocrates (born 406 BC on the Greek island of Cos), known as the 'Father of Medicine'. Encouraged teaching medicine, to act in the best interests of patients and abstain from whatever is deleterious and mischievous, and maintain patient confidentiality.

However the Oath also outlawed abortion and gave emphasis to principles such as paternalism. The original oath is no longer taken in most medical schools.

Helsinki declaration and Geneva declaration: More recent codes developed in response to the atrocities of two world wars. Came about as a result of the Nuremburg War Trials where Nazi doctors were found guilty of conducting experiments on a range of people including Jews, homosexuals, and disabled people. The declarations made recommendations covering both medical practice and research.

Medical school promises: Numerous medical schools worldwide have now developed their own promises based on the Hippocratic Oath and these later declarations, which new doctors take on graduation.

Rights

Some matters are considered to be basic human rights. The Human Rights Act 1998 brought the basic rights outlined in the European Convention on Human Rights into statutory English law. These basic rights include the right to life, right to privacy, right to form a family (and more!) See the website *www.hmso.gov.uk/acts/acts1998* for the full version of the act.

In order to have a right, there is a corresponding duty on others to ensure that this right is not infringed. This means that, for example, you are not allowed to kill someone because this would infringe on their right to life.

The four principles of bioethics

Many of you will be introduced to medical ethics at your medical school through learning 'the four principles'. These are:

- **Autonomy** – the principle of 'self-rule'. People should be allowed to make their own decisions about what happens to them.
- **Beneficence** – do good.
- **Non-maleficence** – this comes from the Latin phrase 'primum non nocere', which means 'above all, do no harm'.
- **Justice** – ensuring that people are treated fairly and equally.

These principles, coined by two American philosophers Beauchamp and Childress, are a way in which you can structure your thoughts when you are first faced with ethical situations. They enable you to give initial consideration as to how best to deal with problems. However, there are many other theories that explore further aspects of philosophy. By using the four principles in combination with some of these other ideas, you will be able to give a more complete argument and therefore address ethical problems more effectively.

Paternalism

A form of doctor-patient relationship. Doctors act as the patient's 'parent' and tell them what to do, even making choices on their behalf. Fortunately this behaviour is less common nowadays, and has been replaced to a greater or lesser degree by respect for patient autonomy.

Utilitarianism/consequentialism

Developed by John Stuart Mill in the 19th century, stating that the correct action is that which gives the 'greatest good for the greatest number'. This requires calculating outcomes and the predicted benefit that they will provide for both individuals and society.

Kantianism/deontology

Counter-argument to utilitarianism. **Immanuel Kant** was a Prussian philosopher in the 18th century. He said that some things are just 'right' – he defines all kinds of 'rights' and 'wrongs'. He stated that you should never treat people as a means to an end, but always as an 'end in themselves'. In other words, you should never subject a human being to anything that isn't 'right', even if the result is that many more people will benefit.

Narrative ethics

Takes peoples' lives in their individual context into account when determining what is ethically correct and incorrect. Dismisses rules and principles.

LEGAL

British judicial system

Cases may enter at any 'level' of court. Either party may appeal to a higher court if they are dissatisfied with the judgement.

Throughout the UK, the House of Lords is the highest court in the land for **civil** cases (any case which is not a criminal case) and until relatively recently, its rulings could not be appealed elsewhere. In Scotland, the High Court of Justiciary is the highest court in relation to **criminal** appeals arising from convictions in Scottish courts; these cases **cannot** be appealed to the House of Lords in England.

The European Courts, especially the European Court of Human Rights, are being used more and more as a result of the European Convention on Human Rights. See www.echr.coe.int for further information about this court, which is increasingly used as the court of last resort.

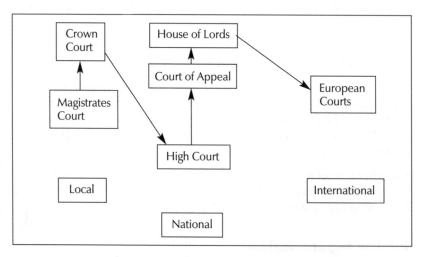

The diagram above shows the organisation of the court system in England and Wales as a general guide to the different levels of the judicial process. This will vary in each jurisdiction and we will not attempt to provide a comprehensive overview here.

Judges

In England and Wales judges in the High Court are called 'Justice' (J). In the Court of Appeal they are 'Lord Justice'(LJ). The House of Lords has five Law Lords (L).

General Medical Council

The General Medical Council (GMC) regulates the UK medical professions, maintains the medical registers of doctors seeking to practise medicine in the UK and provides guidance for practice (e.g. Duties of a Doctor). It has the power to discipline doctors if necessary, and to remove them from the register (which we call 'being struck off').

Historically the British Courts have given substantial power to the GMC in allowing doctors to make decisions about the consequences of poor practice. This is partly because the courts accept that judges are not medically experienced.

Recent trends have involved courts more and more. This may be due to increased awareness and expectations of the public with regard to medical care, coupled with the fact that access to legal services is becoming easier.

Although the GMC is given considerable autonomy in dealing with doctors, although in some cases doctors may be tried by both the GMC and the British legal system.

Common law and statute law

There are two different types of law in the UK. Common law (sometimes known as case law) looks at past cases that have been tested in court. The judgements of these cases become a part of law. This can be superseded in future cases if a judge deems that society considers old rulings to be outdated and no longer appropriate.

The other type of law is statute law, which consists of all the acts that have been passed by Parliament. For example, the Mental Health Act (1983) and the Human Fertilization and Embryology Act (1990).

Tort law and criminal law

An action that has injured someone can be pursued as a criminal and/or a civil (tort) case. A 'tort' is a wrong that has caused damage to somebody, e.g. assault, battery, or through negligence. If the plaintiff wants the defendant to be prosecuted and sent to prison then the case should be heard in criminal courts. If the plaintiff wants compensation for any damage that resulted from the tort then it must be heard in the civil courts. Negligence is the most common form of tort and as Margaret Brazier states in her book *Medicine, Patients and the Law*:

"The function of the tort of negligence is to compensate an individual injured by another's errors, not to adjudicate on a defendant doctor's general competence."

Plaintiffs and defendants

The plaintiff (or claimant) is the person who brings the claim (e.g. the patient who's complaining about their doctor), and the defendant is the person that they're complaining about (e.g. the doctor).

Referencing system

Legal references look complicated! Transcriptions of court proceedings are written in a variety of law reports. When you see a reference that you want to look up, the best thing to do is take it to a law library and find a friendly librarian to show you where the law reports are! Learning all the abbreviations will take forever.

For example, **Bolam v Friern HMC [1957] 2 All ER 118**. This means the plaintiff is a person called Bolam and the defendant is Friern Hospital Management Committee. The ruling can be found in Volume 2 of the *All England Reports of 1957*; page 118.

CHAPTER 4:
THE CASES

HOW TO USE THIS CHAPTER

A variety of cases follow that draw their inspiration from actual events. You may like to attempt answers to these, either individually or in small groups. Medical teachers may wish to use the cases to stimulate discussion of generic ethical or medico-legal issues.

We don't necessarily give any answers to these cases, but that is because sometimes there **are** no right answers – or none that are more right than your own. What this chapter **will** do is give you some key information that you need to know, in terms of laws and important ethical theories. This will help you to be able to reach decisions both within the context of the following cases, and in your own medical practice.

Each case is summarised at the end. Within the cases, points for discussion and revision have been marked with the following symbols:

☆ **Discussion point**

✳ **Revision point**

Most of the cases deal with a range of different issues. If you want to revise particular themes, refer to the list below that shows which cases cover which aspects. This list of themes was drawn up by the Consensus Group of Teachers of Medical Ethics and Law as a core curriculum for UK medical schools. (Consensus Group of Teachers of Medical Ethics and Law in UK Medical Schools. Teaching medical ethics and law within medical education: a model for the UK core curriculum. *Journal of Medical Ethics* 1998; 24:188–192.)

Core content

• Informed consent and refusal of treatment:
Cases: 2, 4, 5, 3, 8, 9, 10, 11, 12, 13, 19

• The clinical relationship: truthfulness, trust, and good communication:
All cases: 1–20

• Confidentiality:
Cases: 1, 4, 7, 10, 12, 14, 15

• Medical research:
Cases: 6, 8, 16

• Human reproduction and the new genetics:
Cases: 8, 14, 16

• Children:
Cases: 4, 5, 8, 11, 14, 15

• Mental disorders and disabilities:
Cases: 3, 4, 12, 13

• Life, death, dying and killing:
Cases: 2, 3, 5, 8, 9, 13, 14, 16

• Vulnerabilities created by the duties of doctors and medical students:
Cases: 3, 5, 6, 7, 8, 10, 13, 14, 15, 18, 20

• Resource allocation:
Cases: 2, 16, 17

• Rights including the Human Rights Act:
Cases: 2, 4, 5, 8, 9, 11, 12, 13, 14, 16, 17, 19

CASE 1: THE DVLA AND THE EPILEPTIC PATIENT

Issues

Driver and Vehicle Licensing Authority (DVLA)
Patient's v society's interests
Breaching confidentiality

You are a recently appointed SpR in neurology. Following investigations during a recent hospital stay, one of your patients, Mr Evans, a middle-aged taxi driver, was diagnosed with epilepsy. Before he left the hospital you advised him to stop driving, and that he should contact the DVLA to make them aware of his diagnosis. Although this meant the end of his livelihood, he undertook to do so.

One month later he is due to attend for an out-patient appointment at your clinic. On the morning of the clinic, one of the specialist nurses (a neighbour of the patient) tells you that he continues to drive. Furthermore, she believes that he has not yet told his wife and family of the diagnosis let alone his employer or the DVLA.

- **What are your responsibilities in this case?**
- **Would you tell:**
  - **The DVLA?**
  - **The family?**
  - **The police?**
  - **The patient?**
  - **The employer?**
- **Should you take any action?**

Use this space to note down your own ideas...

Driver and Vehicle Licensing Authority (DVLA)

It is the patient's responsibility to inform the DVLA of health conditions that might cause them to pose a risk to themselves or other road users by driving. These conditions include:

- Psychiatric disorders e.g. chronic schizophrenia
- Neurological disorders e.g. epilepsy
- Diabetes mellitus
- Visual problems e.g. monocular vision, diplopia

Informing the DVLA does not necessarily lead to automatic suspension – the DVLA will assess whether the condition is severe enough to warrant a driving ban. Certain other medical conditions such as cardiovascular disorders and procedures (e.g. MI or angioplasty) require driving restrictions although the DVLA need not be notified. Doctors should inform their patients if they will need to abstain from driving for a period of time for medical reasons.

If a patient refutes their responsibility and continues to drive then the doctor is morally obliged to take some action. In the first instance you should try to persuade the patient to tell the DVLA himself. In this case, the patient should be persuaded to tell his family the diagnosis too, since it is in his best interests, e.g. they could be educated to provide appropriate care should he have a seizure at home. However, if the patient refuses what can you do?

✳ Doctors are bound by a duty of confidentiality that covers any information they acquire in their professional capacity.

☆ What is confidentiality? What does it mean to the patient? What does it mean to you as a doctor?

Telling the DVLA constitutes a breach of the patient's confidentiality.

☆ On what ethical grounds could you justify such action?

Patient's versus society's interests

In order to **legally** justify breaching confidentiality, not doing so would have to pose a risk to the patient, or to others. In these circumstances the doctor can probably be satisfied that this is the case and is justified in breaching confidentiality.

☆ If this is so, why not just go ahead and tell the DVLA yourself in the first place, instead of depending on a perhaps unreliable patient to do so? What effect would this have on patient care?

☆ If doctors had no code of confidentiality and patients knew that bodies such as the DVLA, insurance companies, the police and the Government could have unlimited access to their health information how would this change medical practice?

☆ What is the point of maintaining patient confidentiality?

☆ In this case, you are told by a third party that the patient is continuing to drive. What happens in situations where you do not have access to such information? How can you be sure the patient will stop driving? How far can/should you go in trying to find out whether they have stopped driving?

Writing to the GP, explaining that you have discussed with the patient the need to inform the DVLA is an obvious first line. Doctors are justified in sharing medical information with other healthcare professionals involved in providing care for their patient. This ensures optimal continuity of care for the patient. It is good practice to always tell the patient that you will write a letter to their GP with any results of investigations done so that you keep them informed. However, patients do have the right to ask that even medical personnel are not told certain information.

☆ Would you be happy to pass the buck to the GP, i.e. assume the GP will make the patient tell the DVLA or, if necessary, tell the DVLA themselves? Do you feel that both you and the GP share this responsibility? Would you feel responsible if the patient caused an accident because he had an epileptic fit while driving?

The GMC gives specific advice in Appendix 2 of its booklet *Confidentiality: Protecting and Providing Information* (Sept 2000).

Breaching confidentiality

If a patient feels that a breach of confidence was not justified they can make a complaint. Although the patient also has the right to take legal action, this can be costly and may not result in the award of any monetary compensation even if the court finds in favour of the plaintiff. If the GMC determined that the doctor was not justified in breaching patient confidentiality, then the doctor could be liable for professional misconduct in the most serious cases and could be struck off the medical register.

The GMC details several possible situations that would allow a doctor to disclose patient information. (GMC, *Confidentiality: Protecting and Providing Information Sept 2000.*) The areas are summarised below:

- If the patient gives written consent e.g. for research
- In the patient's best interests: Sharing information with others providing

care. This includes other healthcare professionals but may exception-
ally, also include a close relative
* In the public interest:
  * if required to do so by a court order or Act of Parliament e.g. notifiable diseases
  * if failure to breach poses a risk of death or serious harm to the patient
or others e.g. child abuse, rape, serious violence

Although the law is broadly in agreement with GMC guidance, the legal
standpoint is less clearly defined. Legally, doctors are justified in breaching
confidentiality **without** the patient's consent in the following circumstances:

* When ordered to do so by law:
  * by a court order
  * under Acts of Parliament e.g. in the case of notifiable diseases
* When it is in the public interest

Breaching confidentiality 'in the public interest' is a very difficult decision to
make and may ultimately be down to the courts to determine. In an English
case (*Hill v Chief Constable for West Yorkshire* [1987] 2 WLR 1126) it was
decided that there was no duty to inform in the public interest.

However, a different view was taken in a famous US case (*Tarasoff v Regents
of the University of California*, Supreme Court of Calif. Sup. 131, Rptr 14 (1
July 1976)). A male college student told a university psychiatrist that he
wanted to kill a fellow student (Tatiana Tarasoff) who had been refusing his
advances. The doctor informed the police, who assessed the situation but
did not make any other intervention. The male student then went ahead
and murdered Tarasoff on her return to campus from holiday.

The parents sued the university for not informing their daughter of the risk.
The US court found the doctor liable for negligence because he had not
warned Tatiana of the potential risk to her life.

In the UK it is unlikely that a similar decision would have been reached
since the doctor took the appropriate action of informing the police. UK
courts are reluctant to make one person liable for the crime committed by
another.

The GMC requires that confidentiality should be maintained even after the
patient's death (see Section 5 of GMC, *Confidentiality: Protecting and
Providing Information Sept 2000*); the law, on the other hand, may not
require this. Note that solicitors and police officers have no special right to
confidential information. Disclose information only if you decide that it is
justified under one of the above conditions.

Breaching confidentiality to relatives

Disclosing information to relatives is sometimes difficult to judge. If it can be assumed that the patient would give consent for information to be disclosed to their family, the doctor can probably go ahead and impart information to the relatives without consulting the patient, who may be either too sick or unable to communicate. However, if the patient has expressly forbidden such communication, this wish should be respected. The patient has a right to maintain confidentiality, even when the doctor considers it not to be in the patient's best interests. Therefore, in the case of the epileptic driver, it may well be in his best interests for his family to know his diagnosis, but if he states that he does not want them to know, you cannot tell them.

Conditions when doctors are legally required to breach confidentiality

- If required to do so by a court of law. Judges will do their best to ensure that any breaches of confidentiality are kept to those relevant to the trial:
  - doctors can be subpoenaed (ordered) to give evidence in court
  - doctors (unlike lawyers) may not refuse to answer questions or withhold evidence
- Prevention of Terrorism Act 1989
  - doctors (like any member of the public) must take the initiative to inform the police of any information regarding terrorist activities
- Police and Criminal Evidence Act 1984
  - doctors must answer police questions or provide any evidence requested by them
  - police can have access to medical records but must abide by certain conditions
- The Public Health (Control of Disease) Act 1984
  - notifiable diseases include cholera, plague, smallpox, relapsing fever, and typhus (N.B. HIV/AIDS is not a notifiable disease)
  - other diseases can fall under this Act should an epidemic occur
- Accidents at work
- Incidents of food poisoning
- Life events:
  - doctors must report births, deaths and abortions
- Misuse of Drugs Act
  - doctors must report details of known drug addicts
- Health Administration:
  - doctors must provide information on request to the Department of Health, regional and district health authorities among others

☆ Can you see any discrepancies in these conditions? It has been argued that people with HIV will be deterred from seeking medical treatment if it is a notifiable disease and that it is therefore not in the public interest to make it notifiable. However, details of drug users must be reported.

If the doctor knows that a patient has, or is about to, commit a criminal offence, they are under no legal obligation to contact the police or provide evidence. The exception to this rule is if the information pertains to terrorist activities. Section 18 of the Prevention of Terrorism Act 1989 states anyone (including doctors) in possession of such information must take the initiative to disclose it to the police. However, if the police contact the doctor, the doctor must answer their questions and provide evidence if necessary under the Police and Criminal Evidence Act 1984.

It could be argued that all citizens have a moral duty to society to prevent and report any crime. The law is excusing doctors from this duty because it believes that there may be situations when it can be in the public interest for doctors to maintain patient confidentiality rather than for certain criminals to be convicted.

If in doubt, seek legal advice from your defence organisation!

Case 1 Summary
- Doctors are bound by a duty of confidentiality to their patients.
- Deciding whether to breach confidentiality requires a careful balance of risk of harm to the patient versus risk of harm to others.
- The law requires doctors to breach confidentiality in certain situations.
- It is the patient's responsibility to inform bodies such as the DVLA or their employer but if the patient refuses, the doctor must take action.

CASE 2: WITHDRAWAL OF VENTILATION

Issues

Advance directives
Consent
'Do not attempt resuscitation' orders
Quality of life issues
Withdrawal of life-saving treatment and the doctrine of the 'Double Effect'
Recent case of Diane Pretty
Communication issues within the healthcare team
Allocation of resources

You are an SHO working in general medicine. A 19-year-old man was diagnosed with motor neurone disease when he was 17. The disease was very aggressive and rapidly progressive.

At a time when his communication was already limited he made it known that he wished to state in an advance directive that should he suffer a cardio-pulmonary arrest he would not want to be resuscitated.

He did suffer a respiratory arrest and was ventilated. You were part of the crash team that attended him. The nurses on the ward did inform the team leader of the advance directive but were told not to interfere.

- **Would you have resuscitated and ventilated this man?**
- **What do you do now that he is on a ventilator?**

Use this space to note down your own ideas…

Advance directives

Advance directives (or living wills) are documents in which a person states the circumstances under which they would and would not wish to receive medical treatment (or to what extent they would want to receive active treatment). This is if and when a situation arises where they are not competent to make their own decisions.

In discussing this case, one would probably look at the situation that the patient was in when the advance directive was made, and consider the validity of that directive.

☆ How do **you** feel about advance directives? What are their pros and cons? Should they be legally binding?

☆ Would you be happy to act according to an advance directive if an unconscious patient was brought in to you? Does your answer to this depend on when the directive was written? If so, do you think they should have an 'expiry date'?

The UK courts have confirmed that a person's advance refusal of treatment should be respected. (*Re T (Adult: refusal of treatment)* [1992] 4 All ER 649; [1992] WLR 782). This depends, however, upon the 'consent' or 'refusal' being valid.

☆ What do you think should be required to ensure that consent is valid?

Consent

In order to be considered valid, consent should be voluntary, informed, and made by a competent individual. There is a case law ruling that consent given by a patient who may have been coerced or under duress to make a certain decision is **not** valid (*Re T (Adult: Refusal of Treatment)* [1992] 4 All ER 649; [1992] WLR 782). Consent is considered to be 'informed' when the patient has received relevant information necessary to make a decision. This includes details of common side effects and risks, as well as potential benefits.

☆ How much do you think you ought to tell someone about a procedure to ensure that they give informed consent? Think about the following procedures:

- Taking blood
- Doing a chest x-ray
- Performing an endoscopy/bronchoscopy
- Performing a vasectomy

Types of consent

Consent can be verbal or written, and it can be explicit or implied. In other words, if somebody rolls up their sleeve and holds their arm out when you ask to take a blood sample, this is implied consent, which is just as good as them saying 'I give consent for you to take my blood'. Note that a signed consent form does not **prove** that a patient gave informed consent, it only **proves** that they signed their name on the form. Therefore, when obtaining a patient's consent, the goal is **not** to get the form signed but to ensure the patient gives informed consent.

Capacity for consent

The law is pretty clear that a person's valid consent or refusal of treatment should be respected. However, in order to give 'valid' consent, a person must have 'capacity', or 'competence' to make decisions.

☆ What do you consider to be important factors in determining a patient's competence to give consent?

British courts considered this matter in a case about a man who suffered from schizophrenia, who was an inpatient at Broadmoor Prison Hospital (*Re C (Adult: Refusal of treatment)* [1994] 1 All ER 819, [1994] 1 WLR 290, [1994] 1 FLR 31, 15 BMLR 77).

The man, C, developed gangrene on two of his toes. His consultant surgeon believed he required a below-the-knee amputation to save his life. The surgeon felt that C's chances of survival without amputation were about 15%, but C stated that he would prefer to die with two feet than live with one. The courts considered whether the mental illness sufficiently reduced C's capacity to understand the nature, purpose and effect of the proposed amputation, therefore making his refusal invalid.

The test described by the High Court in determining an adult's capacity to give consent was:

✳ Can the patient:

- take in and retain treatment information
- believe the information
- weigh that information, balancing risks and needs?

The judge decided that despite his mental illness, C was able to do all of the above, therefore making his refusal of consent valid. In the absence of treatment C's gangrenous toes fell off by themselves and his health was not otherwise affected.

☆ Considering the 'Re C test' in the present case, think about whether the patient would have been competent to give consent at the time he made his feelings known.

We know that the patient in this case had impaired ability to communicate due to his motor neurone disease, but we are not given any information as to his mental capacity.

☆ This patient's condition was described as 'aggressive and rapidly progressive'. Do you think that time could have been a factor in his emotional state and therefore affected his ability to make a competent decision on his views on resuscitation?

Prisoners and consent

☆ Do you think prisoners should be given autonomy? Should they be able to give consent and decide what happens to them, or should this right be removed?

This has been tested in English common law (*Freeman v. Home Office* [1984] All ER 1035, [1984] 2 WLR). A prisoner serving a life sentence claimed that he was unable to give consent. The initial ruling affirmed this idea, but the Court of Appeal later amended the decision and ruled that you should always consider the facts of the case as to whether consent can be valid before accepting it. For example, if a doctor has the power to influence a patient's situation and decision, that patient's consent may not be valid. This could happen in all cases, not just those involving prisoners.

Prisoners are able to give consent, the same as anybody else. The validity of the consent must, however, be certain before it is acted upon.

See Case 4 for a summary of competence.

'Do Not Attempt Resuscitation' (DNAR) orders

Decisions regarding the 'resuscitation status' of patients in hospitals are essentially advance directives. These should, ideally, be made following discussion together with the patient, but this is often not possible. In cases where the patient is not competent to make a decision, it is the responsibility of the doctor in charge of the patient's care to act in the best interests of the patient. Often relatives are involved in situations where patients are incompetent.

☆ Sometimes DNAR orders are assigned to competent patients without their knowledge. Is this right? What happens where you work?

☆ Sometimes DNAR orders are **withheld** from patients in situations even where resuscitation would **not** be in their best interests, simply because their son/daughter is a medical professional or other hospital employee.

Should this have any effect on the care that a patient receives? Whose best interests are at heart in such circumstances?

☆ Do you think that relatives should be able to make decisions on the resuscitation status of a patient? Why/why not? Imagine what it would be like to have a relative who is unconscious in hospital. Remember the need for a doctor to consider the patient's best interests and think about the wider situation of the patient's surroundings when you consider their 'best interests'. For example, how does the involvement and well-being of the family affect the patient? Will it help the patient get better if they have strong family support?

☆ Can you imagine a situation where the relatives may not have the best interests of the patient at the forefront of their minds? Although most relatives are good judges of what patients would want, this is not always the case.

The only way that a relative of an adult patient can make official decisions on medical treatment is if they have 'Durable Power of Healthcare Attorney'. (Definition: Durable Power of Healthcare Attorney can be given to an individual when a patient feels that they may not, in the near future, be able to make their own decisions about medical treatment. Once a person has been given this power of attorney in areas where this is given legal recognition, they make decisions as a 'proxy.')

This has not achieved a status of legal recognition in England, Wales and Northern Ireland, although in Scotland adults may appoint a 'proxy decision-maker' and in many parts of the United States, legislation has given decisions of such people binding force.

(Definition: A proxy decisionmaker is somebody who makes a person's decisions on their behalf. This occurs in England and Wales with medical treatment for children, in which case the parent or legal guardian is able to make 'proxy' decisions.)

Quality of life issues

It is an important part of any decision that a doctor makes in the 'best interests of the patient' to consider the quality of life that would result from any treatment that is administered. Saving somebody's life is not necessarily what the patient would want, as was demonstrated by the wishes of the man in this case. Putting his competence to make decisions aside, he was evidently thinking that life on an artificial ventilator would not be the kind of life that he would want to live. So often in medicine the philosophy of 'active treatment' means that care providers want to do everything they can to help their patients, and it may be difficult for them to accept that sometimes the best thing to do is actually nothing.

Withdrawal of life-saving treatment and the doctrine of the 'Double Effect'

☆ Consider this question: Is the discontinuation of life-saving treatment any different from not initiating the treatment in the first place? Or do you consider it to be more on a par with euthanasia?

The debate of 'stopping' vs. 'not starting' is often considered to be an example of the 'doctrine of the double effect'. This is an ethical term used in situations where one action may have two possible outcomes. For example, sometimes when morphine is used to relieve pain in terminal care the doses prescribed have the side effect of hastening death. The intention is to give pain relief, but there is a 'double effect'. Some people feel that, as long as the intention is to treat pain and not to kill, this is acceptable. However there are also those who believe that the intention is not important – if death is hastened it is not acceptable.

Similarly, views about withdrawing treatment differ. Some argue that withdrawing treatment is no different from not starting treatment in the first place, while others believe that once treatment has started, withdrawing it is equal to euthanasia.

☆ Thinking about withdrawing treatment. What do you consider to be 'treatment' and what do you think is a basic requirement of life? Are the following treatments or fundamental to life?

- antibiotics to treat infection (where the primary diagnosis is cancer)
- intravenous fluids
- tube feeding.

Issues surrounding the withdrawal of treatment are discussed in detail in the case of Tony Bland, a football supporter who was left in a persistent vegetative state following the Hillsborough Disaster in 1989. The case was eventually passed to the House of Lords (*Airedale NHS Trust v Bland* [1993] 1 All ER 521; AC879).

In this case, Lord Goff stated that where a patient lacks capacity, a treatment can be discontinued where its use is no longer considered to be in the patient's best interests.

(Read the judgement of Lord Goff of Chieveley in the Bland case, as it provides a detailed analysis of the ethics and law surrounding this difficult and complicated issue.)

The difficulty for the doctor lies in assessing the best interests of the incompetent patient. New guidance from the GMC (GMC, *Withholding and withdrawing life-prolonging treatments*, August 2002) is useful to refer to.

However, should the patient be competent to make decisions for themselves, they would be able to say whether they wanted the treatment to continue. It is unusual, though not impossible, for a patient who is receiving artificial ventilation to be conscious and competent to decide the future use of the ventilator. One situation where this could feasibly occur is in the case of motor neurone disease, where patients may be of sound mind. In such cases, the patient may be able to pull the tube out, therefore removing their own treatment. Other patients may be unable to move enough to do that. They could well be capable of deciding that they don't want the ventilator, but they would need help in the physical action of removing the equipment.

So if you thought that this patient's advance directive was valid in the first instance, you may consider it right to stop the ventilation. Or if he turned out to regain consciousness and capacity after the arrest incident, he may ask you to remove the tube. If you were the doctor in charge and you considered that the advance directive was invalid, but that continuation of artificial ventilation was no longer in the man's best interests, you may decide to remove the treatment.

Recent case of Dianne Pretty

The recent case of a 43-year-old lady with motor neurone disease may have crossed your mind when discussing the above situation (*R (on the application of Pretty)* v *Director of Public Prosecutions* [2002] FLR 268). It may be worth considering that in this lady's case she was not asking for any treatment to be removed. She was saying that she wanted to commit suicide and because she was unable to perform the act of putting pills in her mouth and swallowing them, or performing any other act of suicide, she was asking the courts to allow her husband to help her do what she would otherwise do by herself. The House of Lords ruled that, despite the patient's competence and autonomy she was asking for her husband to perform an act of assisted suicide, which is not legal in this country.

☆ Do you agree with the House of Lords' ruling in the case of Dianne Pretty? Or would you have allowed her husband to help her to die?

☆ Diane Pretty took her case to the European Court of Human Rights where she ultimately lost her battle. Why do you think this was? (*Case of Pretty v United Kingdom* Application no. 00002346/02. Reference no. REF00003580. See the European Court of Human Rights website www.hudoc.echr.coe.int)

Ironically, the verdict was delivered just a few hours before the UK High Court granted another 43-year-old woman, known as 'Miss B', the right to die. (*Re B (Adult: Refusal of Medical Treatment* [2002] 2 All ER 449).

The crucial difference between the two cases was that Miss B was asking for a treatment to be stopped (a ventilator switched off), whereas Diane Pretty was requesting an intervention to help her to die. Is there an ethical difference between these two actions if the intention and the outcome are the same?

Diane Pretty died in May 2002, two weeks after the ruling, after 10 days of pain and breathing difficulties. She said of the court decisions: "The law has taken all my rights away."

Communication issues within the healthcare team

In this situation the nurse on the ward told the arrest team leader that the patient had signed an advance directive. This raises some important issues about communication and the importance of note-keeping and keeping accurate records of actions in healthcare.

☆ Should it be the responsibility of the nurse looking after a patient to ensure that cardiac arrest teams are not called if the patient suffers an arrest? What about agency nurses and bank staff or healthcare assistants? Should they be expected to know whether to call the team, or is it better for them to make the call and then cancel it? If you are a doctor on the cardiac arrest team and you are the first to arrive at the scene, should it be up to you to check the patient notes to find out if they are meant to be resuscitated, or should you start until somebody tells you otherwise?

Allocation of resources

Resources are always limited in healthcare, and as a result rationing decisions have to be made all the time. A patient who is successfully resuscitated following a cardiac arrest is usually transferred to an ICU for further treatment. Beds in intensive care units are always in short supply, as well as presenting a huge cost to the health service.

☆ If a patient does not wish to be resuscitated if they suffer a cardiac arrest, should the limited resources and funding influence the decision about whether or not to respect their wishes?

Case 2 Summary

- In UK law a person's advance refusal of treatment should be respected.
- **Valid** consent is voluntary, informed, and made by a competent individual.
- Capacity to give consent is specific to individual decisions, and can be assessed using a legal test.
- In England and Wales people may not appoint a legal power of healthcare attorney to make proxy decisions.
- In situations where patients are not competent to give consent, doctors may treat if it is in the best interests of the patient.

CASE 3: THE INCOMPETENT ADULT AND ADVANCE DIRECTIVES

Issues

Advance directives
Relatives
Proxy consent and the Adults with Incapacity Act (Scotland) 2000
The law on euthanasia in The Netherlands: recent developments

Sue is a 56-year-old solicitor. She becomes aware that her memory is deteriorating rapidly and her grasp of what is going on around her is loosening. She is diagnosed as suffering from early onset of Alzheimer's Disease. While at this stage, she completes an advance directive in consultation with her GP, a family friend.

Nine months later, the disease has progressed rapidly, to the extent that Sue no longer recognises her immediate family. Following a bout of flu, she is admitted to hospital with suspected pneumonia.

Her husband Donald says she should not be given an antibiotic, in accordance with her advance directive. He says this was exactly the situation she had contemplated while still able to express her wishes.

Sue's 35-year-old daughter Sally is vigorously insisting that you pull out all the stops and treat her mother as you would any other patient with a respiratory infection.

- **Do you give her antibiotics?**
- **What influences your decision?**

Use this space to note down your own ideas…

Advance directives

✳ Remember that in the UK an advance refusal of treatment is respected provided that the initial directive was valid.

☆ How can you be sure that Sue's advance directive still represents her present views?

Relatives

The views held by a patient's relatives can have a substantial influence over the care that a patient receives. Legally, in England and Wales, relatives have very few rights in determining medical care, however good medical practice recognises that there are in fact several 'patients' in most medical cases. The emotional and psychological effects suffered by relatives who are not kept as informed as they would like, or who perhaps feel that their loved one is not being treated in the way that they would like to see, can be massive.

It is a doctor's duty to act in accordance with the wishes and best interests of the patient. If this involves going against the ideals, attempts may be made to discuss the issue with the relatives with the aim of reaching a mutual agreement.

In this case Sue's daughter insists that you 'treat her mother as you would any other patient with a respiratory infection'.

☆ How might you consider discussing the issue with Sue's daughter?

☆ Would you explain that you are treating Sue according to her own wishes?

☆ Would you tell the daughter that it is not uncommon for patients who are very unwell not to receive antibiotics? Antibiotics are potent drugs with many side effects. If these side effects cause substantial discomfort (e.g. diarrhoea) and outweigh any potential benefits they may not be considered appropriate.

☆ What else would you try to discuss? Is there anything you would not want to talk about?

Proxy consent and the Adults with Incapacity Act (Scotland) 2000

☆ What do you think about relatives giving consent on behalf of patients? What are the potential benefits of this? Can you imagine any possible problems that may arise?

The Adults with Incapacity Act (Scotland) has now made it legal to give or withhold consent on behalf of other adults in Scotland. The Act covers affairs relating to the property, finances and welfare of 'incapable adults'.

The welfare part of the Act, which relates to medical treatment, came into force from 1 July 2002. Under the Act, 'incapacity' is defined as:

- incapable of acting; or
- making decisions; or
- communicating, understanding or remembering decisions.

This could be due to a mental disorder or an inability to communicate due to physical disability. Most people protected by the Act will have a form of dementia, learning disability or will have suffered an accident or head injury. Capacity is task specific: some patients may be capable to consent to IV hydration but unable to consent to a coronary angioplasty, since the procedure is more complicated.

When faced with an adult who lacks capacity, healthcare workers must make efforts to contact the person who has been designated welfare attorney/ guardian. This is most likely to be the next of kin. The public guardian can be contacted if it is unclear whether the patient has a welfare attorney/ guardian, or if you do not have their contact details.

As a doctor you must make treatment decisions through consultation with the patient's welfare attorney. They should have full access to information, as any **patient** would, so the GMC has changed its guidance regarding breaching confidentiality in this respect.

When you treat an incapable adult you must aim to:

- benefit the adult
- only provide treatment that provides benefit
- choose the least restrictive option
- take into account the past and present wishes and feelings of the adult
- consider views of relevant others.

If the welfare attorney disagrees with the doctor regarding treatment, a second medical opinion should be sought. If there is still disagreement the matter can be taken to court for resolution.

In order to treat an incapable adult, the healthcare professional should complete a form (S47) that details why the adult is incapable in this case and the treatment plan proposed. This can be done in the absence of a welfare attorney if the patient does not have one, but must be completed. The form is valid for the duration of the treatment plan, up to a maximum of 12 months.

Note that this Act does not cover emergency treatment. If an incapable adult requires immediate treatment to save their life or safeguard their health this can be administered without delay.

For more information look at the BMA website www.bma-org.uk.

In England and Wales, although some people believe that the person who they have made their legal power of attorney has the ability to proxy consent, this is not the case.

The law on euthanasia in the Netherlands: recent developments

Maaike Möller BSc (Bioethics), Medical Student, University of Bristol

An explicit policy on euthanasia began to develop in The Netherlands in the early 1970s. At first purely jurisprudential, this policy was officially legalised in 2001. Despite much international attention this legislation was largely symbolic and practice remained relatively unchanged.

The most important discussions currently taking place in The Netherlands centre around the qualifying conditions for euthanasia which have always formed the very core of the policy. These so-called "due care" criteria stipulate that a doctor can only be exempt from prosecution for euthanasia if he/she is satisfied, among other things, that the patient has made a voluntary and well-considered request and that the suffering is unbearable and without prospect of improvement or relief. The act of euthanasia must therefore be both autonomous and beneficent.

Recently, however, two cases in particular have highlighted situations in which there appears to be a conflict between these two principles. In the 1994 Chabot case the Supreme Court ruled that psychiatric suffering may qualify for euthanasia under the 'due care' criteria. Currently, the Brongersma case (2000 and 2001) is causing controversy on the matter of whether or not the 'life fatigue' of very elderly people who are simply 'finished with living' might similarly constitute suffering so unbearable as to qualify for euthanasia under the criteria.

On the one hand, if suffering is to be considered as subjective, if a person wishes to die their pain must almost by definition be such that it is 'unbearable' according to the 'due care' criteria.

On the other hand, the implications of the acceptance of non-medical suffering within euthanasia are potentially extremely significant. The medicalisation of all suffering changes notions of 'illness' and subsequently the role of the doctor. It might also increase fear of all suffering and that associated with old age in particular.

The Brongersma case – a summary

Edward Brongersma was a former senator and prominent public figure who, aged 86, was 'tired of life' and felt that 'death had forgotten him'.

He had repeatedly asked his general practitioner, Philip Sutorius, to assist him in his suicide and in April 1998 his request was granted. The public prosecutor consequently instigated criminal proceedings against Sutorius on the grounds that he did not adhere to one of the 'due care' criteria, namely that the suffering should be unbearable and without prospect of relief.

In October 2000 the District Court of Haarlem acquitted Sutorius on the basis of expert testimony on the subjectivity of suffering. The public prosecutor appealed against the verdict. In November 2001, on the basis of the testimony of two experts who had been asked to investigate the case, the Court of Appeal in Amsterdam convicted Sutorius of violating the 'due care' criteria. The court judged that 'life fatigue' is a general social, rather than a specifically medical, problem and it should therefore not be considered under the 'due care' criteria of the euthanasia policy. The discussion on the matter is, however, far from over.

Case 3 Summary

- Although legally a patient's relatives have very few rights in medical decision making, good medical practice requires you to balance relatives' legal rights with the fact that they themselves may need your help and advice.
- New law in Scotland (the Adults with Incapacity Act 2000) makes it possible to make decisions on behalf of other adults. This covers various decisions including those on medical treatment.
- Doctors in the Netherlands can be exempt from prosecution for euthanasia if they satisfy strict criteria.

CASE 4: THE 16-YEAR-OLD DIABETIC

Issues

Duty of care
Good Samaritan acts
Refusing treatment
Competence and age of medical consent

You are an SHO in A&E. Daniel, a 16-year-old male, is brought to your department by his school friends. They say that he is acting "weird …drunk-like." They claim he has not been drinking and does not use drugs; they have spent the afternoon skateboarding in the sunshine. They then depart.

Daniel is brought through to a cubicle and is seen by the triage nurse. His speech is slurred, his movements are unco-ordinated; he is aggressive and refuses treatment: "I just wanna get out of here… . Leave me alone you bastards, don't you dare touch me." While the nurse goes to find you, he runs from the hospital leaving behind his school bag. You look inside his bag to check for an address, and find vials of insulin and some sugar sachets, as well as his home address.

- **What do you do next?**
- **Do you have a continuing duty of care now that he has left the hospital?**
- **Who would you contact? Should you talk to:**
  - **his parents/guardians**
  - **his school**
  - **the police**
- **If he had been 15 would it have made a difference?**

Use this space to note down your own ideas…

Duty of care

Hospitals which have no A&E department are not legally obliged to assume a duty of care for patients that turn up on its doorstep. However, the hospital in this case has an A&E department which means it is prepared to assume a duty of care for anyone turning up at the hospital. Your duty of care started when he entered the hospital, and without proper assessment of the situation you cannot discharge that duty simply because he left the department.

You know very little about this patient. There are several possible explanations for his behaviour:

- he may be hypo- or hyper-glycaemic
- he may be drunk or on drugs, even though his friends have said this is not the case
- he may have nothing wrong with him at all and just be playing around.

There is a real chance that he may be hypo- or hyper-glycaemic. You should suspect this because of the way in which he was brought in and because you found the insulin in his bag. There is therefore the possibility that he may require medical attention and you should make efforts to deliver this.

To try to track him down there are several options open to you. If you ask the police to help to find him you do not have to divulge anything more about him other than that he needs medical attention. However, it is always best to tell the police your concerns as fully as possible so that they can help in the most appropriate way, i.e. not treat him as a dangerous criminal. As part of their search, they will go to his home and contact his parents. The parents may find it more distressing to have the police chasing their son than if they were to hear about the problem through the hospital. For these reasons, it is probably best to contact the parents in the first instance. You will then also be able to build up a fuller history of Daniel that may help to explain his behaviour better.

Bear in mind that when trying to track down patients in this way, you have a duty to respect the patient's confidentiality. However, in this case, you have very little information about Daniel so there is very little you could disclose.

Although he has run away, he may not be aware that he needs to be treated nor of the consequences of refusing treatment. In addition, diabetic teenagers are often in denial about their illness and their need for treatment. You cannot therefore assume that he has competently refused treatment. If Daniel is found and you strongly suspect that his mental state is compromised due to his hypo- or hyperglycaemia, he would be regarded as an incompetent minor. In such cases, at the age of 16, his parents or guardians would be able to consent to treatment on his behalf.

Good Samaritan acts

As a doctor you have no legal obligation to treat people you meet beyond your medical duties. For example, if the captain on an aircraft puts out a call asking if there are any doctors on board, you would not be found negligent in British law if you decided not to volunteer your services (although you may feel a moral duty to assist). However, if you did decide to come forward, you would be assuming a duty of care and could be open to prosecution if things went wrong. It is unlikely that a patient would bring such an action to court, and even more unlikely that a court would find in favour of the plaintiff. It is in society's interests to encourage skilled people to help in emergency situations without the threat of legal action being a deterrent. Some doctors are reluctant to stop at accident sites or offer their services indiscriminately. However, most doctors would have a hard time ignoring such a cry for help.

☆ How would you behave if you came across someone in need of medical attention? Is it ethical to refuse to help? Do you think doctors should be forced to treat in such circumstances?

In some countries, e.g. France and Germany, doctors *are* required to offer assistance when it is called for. Note that if you are in one of these countries or even on board a Lufthansa or Air France aeroplane you would also be required to obey the laws of these countries.

If you are the sort of person who would offer assistance, make sure you are indemnified by a medical defence organisation that covers 'Good Samaritan acts'.

Refusing treatment

Competent patients

As has been discussed in a previous case (Case 2), competent patients aged 18 or over have the right to refuse treatment. Building on the legal test of competence outlined in Case 2, the BMA (Consent Tool Kit, 2001) recommend the following.

✳ A patient is considered competent if he/she is able to:

- understand what the medical treatment is, and why it is being proposed
- understand the main benefits, risks and alternatives
- understand the consequences of not receiving the proposed treatment
- retain the information for long enough to make an effective decision
- make a free choice and not be under pressure.

Incompetent patients

Under 18's

If a patient is aged under 18 years and lacks capacity to consent, a person or local authority with parental responsibility may consent to treatment on their behalf. If the two parents disagree about whether the treatment should be given or not, it may be necessary to take the matter to the courts.

The current legal situation means that the mother automatically has parental responsibility for her child once it is born. If the parents are not married the mother is the only parent who has parental responsibility and therefore the only one who can consent to treatment. This applies unless a written agreement can be arranged whereby the mother agrees that the father can have parental rights.

☆ Is this ethical? How do you feel about an unmarried father's rights?

Over 18's

In England and Wales, incompetent adults (aged 18 or over) cannot have someone else consent to treatment for them (in Scotland it is different – see Case 3). In these cases, doctors are often allowed to treat if it is in the best interests of the patient. In deciding this, it may be wise to consult with relatives to try to learn more about what the patient would have wanted (see Case 5).

☆The law uses age to determine whether or not someone is able to consent to treatment. Is this the best measure of competence? Is it ethical? What happens in cases where a patient has a chronological age of 30 yet a 'mental age' of 4? (See Case 12).

Case 4 Summary

- Doctors have a duty of care to people who they accept as patients.
- Competent patients aged 18 or over have the right to refuse treatment.
- Parents or guardians of incompetent patients under the age of 18 can consent to treatment on the patient's behalf.
- Incompetent patients aged 18 or over can be treated if it is in their best interests.
- Determining what is appropriate in the best interests of a patient requires consultation with relatives and those involved in the care of the patient.

CASE 5: THE 15-YEAR-OLD JEHOVAH'S WITNESS

Issues

Competence under age 16
Refusing treatment – competent minors
Ward of court
Considering 'best interests'

You are a surgical SHO called to A&E for an emergency standby. Sam, a 15-year-old male, is brought in following a road traffic accident. He has been knocked off his bike, resulting in a complicated fracture of his right femur with major blood loss. He requires rapid surgery.

Sam is lucid on admission and clearly states to you: "I am a Jehovah's Witness. Please don't transfuse me. Will you promise to contact my church, doctor?"

You explain the probable consequences of not transfusing, especially due to the amount of blood he has already lost, and the limitations of artificial blood products. However he is adamant that he does not wish to be transfused. Shortly after this exchange, he lapses into unconsciousness.

The charge nurse finds an identity card in his wallet confirming that Sam is a Jehovah's Witness, and would refuse a blood transfusion if it were required. You are asked not to contact the Jehovah's Witness church elders.

- **What should you do next?**
- **May you go ahead and operate, transfusing as necessary, thereby overriding Sam's express wishes?**
- **Should your hospital apply to have this patient made a ward of court? If so, why?**
- **Regardless of whether you intend to go ahead and transfuse Sam, should you contact his church as per his request?**

Use this space to note down your own ideas...

Competence under age 16

Age 16 is the age of medical consent. It is assumed that people aged 16 or over have the necessary capacity to give valid consent to treatment. However, if a person under that age can demonstrate that they are competent to give consent (See Case 4) this can be taken as valid. Although parental involvement should be encouraged, if a competent person requests that matters are kept confidential this wish should be respected.

The Gillick case

The phrase 'Gillick competence' has become part of common language in the last 15 years. It is useful to know how it came about and what it actually means.

In 1982 Mrs Victoria Gillick, then the mother of four girls under the age of 16, was concerned that her daughters may be given contraceptive and abortion advice or treatment without her knowledge or consent. She went to court to try to ensure that this would not be allowed to happen. However, her demands were rejected on this initial trial (*Gillick v West Norfolk and Wisbech AHA* [1984] 1 All ER 365).

The judge decided that contraception and abortion advice and treatment are the same as any medical treatment. He decreed that the law must allow competent people under the age of 16 to give valid consent to medical treatment in confidence. It was up to the doctor to decide whether the young person was mature enough to satisfy the conditions of competence.

Mrs Gillick then took her case to the Court of Appeal and won ([1985] 1 All ER 533, CA) The judges overturned the previous decision, stating that parental rights under common law were binding, no matter how mature and independent the young person. Under the age of 16, parents had control over their children and what happened to them, including medical treatment and advice. This implied that doctors could only see or examine a child under 16 with a parent present. The only exception would be in emergency situations, when common law would allow a doctor to treat without waiting for parental consent. The ruling also meant that it became illegal to give information on contraception or abortion to anyone under 16 without parental consent. Sex education in schools could be outlawed under this ruling.

The case was ultimately taken to the House of Lords. It was only by a majority of three to two, that the Law Lords ruled against the Court of Appeal. They decided that parental rights were **necessary** only until the child had reached sufficient intellectual maturity to make her own decisions. Competent people under 16 should be allowed to give valid consent to medical examination and treatment including that relating to contraception and abortion ((1985) 3 All ER 402).

It is ironic that we now use the phrase 'Gillick competent' to describe a competent minor when in fact Mrs Gillick was arguing against the existence of this in principle.

Certain other things arose out of the Gillick case that have had an impact on medical practice.

- Under Section 28 of the Sexual Offences Act 1956, it is an offence to 'cause or encourage ... the commission of unlawful sexual intercourse with ... a girl for whom [the] accused is responsible'. The Law Lords decided that it would not be a criminal offence for a doctor to prescribe contraception for a girl in the best interests of her health. This would not be seen as encouragement if the doctor was sure that without the contraception she would continue to have sex, exposing herself to further risks such as pregnancy, abortion or childbirth.
- However, as Lord Scarman said: 'Clearly a doctor who gives ... [a patient] ... contraceptive advice or treatment not because in his clinical judgement the treatment is medically indicated ... but with the intention of facilitating her having unlawful sexual intercourse may well be guilty of a criminal offence.'(p.425 [1985] 3 All ER 402). It is not clear where the line is drawn between encouraging sexual intercourse and allowing it.

For further discussion of the Gillick case and its issues, go to the law reports referenced in this section or *Medicine, Patients and the Law* by Margaret Brazier.

Refusing treatment – competent minors

We have looked at what happens when minors lack capacity to consent to treatment in Case 4. What happens though, when a **competent** person under the age of 16 actively **refuses** treatment such as in the case of Sam?

Competent minors are able to give consent to treatment in the absence of parental consent, and even in the unlikely situation of the parents actively refusing consent. However, in England and Wales they are not allowed to refuse consent, if the parents (or a court) give their consent. This is like saying that the consent of such minors is only valid if it agrees with the medical opinion. As long as either the minor or someone with parental responsibility gives consent, the procedure can go ahead, regardless of the wishes of the other party.

☆ Do you agree with this? Is this an ethically justifiable position? On what grounds?

It is possible that the implementation of the Human Rights Act may force such cases to be dealt with differently in English law – the wish of a competent minor to refuse treatment could be upheld.

In Scotland the situation is also unclear, but it is likely that the decision of a competent minor to refuse life-saving treatment could *not* be overridden by their parents or by a court.

Ward of court

In such difficult situations it may be best to let the courts decide. If this is what you want to do you should seek legal advice and apply to make the child a 'ward of court'. If the court assumes wardship of the child all decisions on the medical treatment of the child will be made by the court, acting in their best interests.

The issues at stake include the need to balance the harm caused by violating the young person's wishes with the harm caused by failing to treat. In determining the child's best interests it makes perfect sense to contact the church, as Sam has requested, to gather as much information as possible about his beliefs.

If you go ahead and treat Sam you should try to minimise the harm done to him by initially trying alternatives to blood transfusions. There are several alternatives, none as effective as blood, and if they do not work you would have to consider giving him the transfusions.

Considering 'best interests'

☆ What factors do you think are important when determining a patient's best interests? Brainstorm a list yourself before looking at the following paragraph.

The BMA has come up with a list of things that need to be considered (British Medical Association, Consent Tool Kit, 2001):

- The patient's own wishes and values, including any advance statement
- Clinical judgement about the effectiveness of the proposed treatment, particularly in relation to other options
- Where there is more than one option, which option is least restrictive of the patient's future choices
- The likelihood and extent of any degree of improvement in the patient's condition if treatment is provided

- The views of the parents, if the patient is a child
- The views of people close to the patient, especially close relatives, partners, carers or proxy decisionmakers about what the patient is likely to see as beneficial
- Any knowledge of the patient's religious, cultural and other non-medical views that might have an impact on the patient's wishes.

None of these aspects on its own can determine the final decision, and all should be taken into account.

Case 5 Summary

- Patients aged 16 years or older can give consent to medical treatment.
- Patients under 16 can give consent if they demonstrate that they are competent to do so.
- When a competent patient under 16 refuses consent, doctors can consult with their parents/guardians and the courts if necessary. Treatment may go ahead if it is in the best interests of the patient but this needs to be carefully considered.
- Common Law covers emergency situations: doctors can treat patients immediately in situations where it is assumed that consent would be given and if the delay required to obtain consent would cause serious harm to the patient.

CASE 6: THE NEGLIGENT SURGEON

Issues

Negligence
Reporting poor clinical practice
Doctors and their families requiring medical treatment

You are an SHO working in A&E. You have noticed that since you started four months ago you have seen several female patients who show signs of sepsis, significant post-operative bleeding and unsightly surgical scars. All of these women have been operated on by Ms Smith, and their complications appear to be a direct result of the surgery. You know Ms Smith well, as she is a very popular surgeon with patients, nurses and doctors alike.

You overhear two theatre sisters discussing that Ms Smith is getting a bit shaky. You suspect that her lack of technical skill is causing harm to her patients – who you then have to see in A&E to pick up the pieces. Your mother is due to have a hysterectomy in six weeks' time under Ms Smith.

- **Do you tell:**
  - **your educational supervisor in A&E?**
  - **a consultant colleague of Ms Smith in Obs and Gynae?**
  - **your friend, an SHO in Obs and Gynae?**
  - **Ms Smith?**
  - **your mother?**
- **Regardless of whether you decide to tell your mother, do you try to make sure your mother's hysterectomy is carried out by another surgeon?**

Use this space to note down your own ideas…

Negligence

✳ A doctor can be found negligent due to failure to:

- make a correct diagnosis
- treat; or failure to
- warn of risks involved in a procedure or treatment.

If a patient believes that a doctor's performance in one of these areas is inadequate, they may initiate claims procedures for negligence.

✳ To do this, they must prove that the:

- doctor owed them a duty of care (see Case 10)
- doctor's standard of care was less than should be expected by a reasonable doctor in that post
- negligence caused them injury which they would otherwise not have sustained.

The burden of proof in negligence cases lies with the plaintiff (i.e. the patient). This makes it difficult for patients to succeed in negligence claims.

Reporting poor clinical practice

Ever since the Bristol Heart Case, where large numbers of operations were performed on children with sub-optimal results, legislation and professional codes have been put into place whereby poor clinical practice can (and should) be reported without the person who 'blows the whistle' being reprimanded.

Since the 'Whistle Blowing Act' was passed (see Case 19), the Government has created a structure for 'Clinical Governance', through which NHS trusts and employees regulate their progress and continuously audit and evaluate their success to improve practice where necessary. As a direct result of clinical governance, individuals are no longer necessarily held personally responsible when something goes wrong. Instead, the hospital will look at what happened and why, and make changes to ensure that the same mistake is not made a second time.

Doctors and their families requiring medical treatment

☆ Should doctors get preferential treatment on the NHS? For example, do you think they should jump the waiting list? Or should they always see a consultant in clinic, and not a junior doctor?

☆ Should the action that you take regarding your concerns about Ms Smith be affected by the fact that you know your mother is due to be operated on next week?

☆ If you wish to prevent your mother from being operated on by Ms Smith, isn't it ethical to prevent other women from the same fate? Some doctors refer to this logic as the 'granny test': If you would not like your grandmother to be treated in a particular way or by a particular person, no-one else should be subjected to it either. This 'test' could just as easily be called the 'father', 'daughter' or 'best friend' test, depending on the circumstances.

Case 6 Summary

- Negligence can be due to failure to diagnose, treat, or warn of risks involved in treatment.
- Negligence claims can be difficult for patients to win, as the burden of proving that the doctor was negligent lies with the patient.
- A successful negligence claim proves that the defendant had a duty of care, that they did not provide the standard of care expected of the reasonable doctor in that post (i.e. an SHO is compared with SHOs; a consultant compared with consultants), and that the injury in question occurred as a direct result of the negligence.

CASE 7: THE SICK COLLEAGUE

Issues

Looking after each other – ethics for working in a team
Risks to patients
Stealing from the hospital
Breaking the law

You are an SHO in anaesthetics. Late one night, after a 'heavy' hospital Christmas party, Clare, a highly competent and popular junior surgical colleague (a fellow SHO) tells you that she thinks she is Hep C+ve. You have known her since medical school and often work together in theatre.

The next morning you are sitting in the coffee room when one of the surgical staff nurses (a friend of yours) approaches and asks: "Can I have a quiet word?" She is concerned that drugs, particularly diamorphine ampoules, have been going missing from the controlled drugs trolley on her ward. There is as yet unofficial but widespread suspicion among the ward staff that colleague Clare has been taking them. Nobody has done anything yet because of her popularity.

- **What do you say to the theatre nurse?**
- **What are your responsibilities in this case?**
- **Do you discuss the issue with**
  - **Clare?**
  - **another SHO friend?**
  - **your educational supervisor?**
  - **Clare's educational supervisor?**
  - **the GMC?**
  - **no-one?**

Use this space to note down your own ideas...

Looking after each other – ethics for working in a team

The nature of healthcare means that doctors and other healthcare profession-als need to work in teams so that they can deliver the best possible care for patients 24 hours a day. It is essential that everyone is able to work effectively within the team so that this goal can be achieved. It is also important that indi-viduals within the team can ask for and receive support and help from each other when necessary. This is an inherent aspect of working together and directly affects the enjoyment of staff and the quality of patient care. Looking after each other's physical and emotional welfare could include matters like getting coffee or snacks for each other during busy periods, and making sure the workload is fair. It may be necessary occasionally to provide extra support in certain situations and this case illustrates such an example.

The NHS is all about putting the patients' needs first but sometimes this causes the welfare of the staff to be neglected. The irony is that the better the staff are looked after, the better care they will take of the patients. Working in the NHS, and healthcare in general, means that staff are confronted by many different sources of stress. It may not be as easy as it is in other lines of work to create a happy and healthy working environment, but it is possible. Making time to socialise together outside work is a good way to enhance team spirit.

☆ Team members need to be able to trust and respect one another. Do you automatically trust other members of the team or does it take time for you to regard them as worthy of your trust? Why?

☆ Patients often trust doctors simply because they are doctors. What do you think about this? Is this trust usually justified? If it is, should you also auto-matically trust other doctors? If you don't, why don't you?

☆ How do you decide whether you can trust someone? Is there anything you can do or say which will help others (colleagues and patients) to see you as a trustworthy person?

☆ Is it necessary to inform on each other's every mistake or problem? What kind of atmosphere would this create within the workplace? Where do we draw the line i.e. how bad must the problem be?

You should consider how much risk the mistake poses to the welfare of others (patients or staff) and whether it is a risk that is constantly present, likely to occur again or a one-off incident.

Looking after each other means taking action to help each other within the goal of protecting patients. It does not mean 'protecting' each other in such a way that would jeopardise patient care.

The GMC has specific guidance about working with colleagues and encourages problems to be initially dealt with within the team. This may mean speaking to the colleague directly, or asking another team member or senior to become involved. Occasionally, it may be necessary to seek help from outside the team, e.g. the Trust medical director, or the GMC.

A colleague who is taking drugs or carrying a serious communicable disease may present a risk to patients. You have a moral duty to protect patients from such risks so you must take action. The question is, what type of action? You must decide at what level you think the problem is best handled. Think about the following issues when making your decision.

Risks to patients

Drug abuse

The first question you must ask is whether the drug abuse affects the doctor's ability to care for patients. If you believe it does, or it could, you must act quickly.

You should make every effort to find out the facts in this situation. If you have a close relationship with this person it may be possible for you to discuss the issues with them. Remember that drug users can be so addicted to the drug that it changes their personality, causing them to lie or steal to keep their habit, when normally they would have never done such things.

If the colleague is a friend of yours and they are able to discuss their problem with you sensibly, this is a good start. You can help your colleague while protecting patients at the same time. If the colleague acknowledges the risk they are taking with their own health and the health of patients, they should agree to take some time off and get help. If there is a senior person with whom the colleague feels able to discuss the problem, this may help. The employer and/or GMC may ultimately need to be informed, and this is best done by the colleague themselves.

Things become more difficult if the colleague denies the problem or refuses to recognise the risk to patients. This is when a senior member of staff should be involved. If there is no such person around, e.g. in the case of a GP who is working single-handed, it may be necessary to contact the employer and/or GMC yourself. The GMC has the power to remove doctors from the medical register if it decides they are unfit to practise medicine or pose a risk to patients. Abusing drugs is regarded as 'serious professional misconduct'.

Other issues to think about:

☆ What do you define as a 'drug'? Does it matter what type of drug is being used? Are illegal drugs morally or legally different to legal drugs such as alcohol? Is there a difference between someone who uses cocaine while off duty and someone who gets drunk while off duty?

☆ Is your ability to care for patients affected if you have not slept enough or are too tired? There was a recent court case where a tired driver was convicted of manslaughter and sent to prison. He had fallen asleep at the wheel and accidentally drove onto a railway track. He caused multiple deaths when a train crashed into his car (Selby rail crash. The driver was convicted on 10 counts of causing death by dangerous driving in December 2001, and sentenced to five years in prison in January 2002). It is possible that a doctor could be found negligent for making a mistake because he was tired. In such cases however, patients are more likely to take court action against the hospital for forcing the doctor to work such long hours. Hospitals and doctors are taking action to reduce working hours and if you are being forced to work unreasonable/illegal amounts of time you should take the issue up with your employer and the BMA.

✳ Note that any mistake by a doctor, whether or not their ability is diminished by drugs or alcohol, may result in the doctor being found negligent in law (see Case 6).

Even if you believe the colleague does not present a risk to patients you may still want to discuss things with them. Maybe there is an underlying reason for their behaviour, such as depression. Be aware that the medical profession has a high incidence of depression, suicide and divorce. How would you feel if a colleague committed suicide? By helping to create a climate of mutual care within the team you can also be confident of the support of your colleagues should you ever need it yourself.

Risk-taking in general

☆ What do you think about people who use drugs?

☆ How do you treat patients who you know are drug abusers? How should you treat them?

☆ Do you feel a patient with endocarditis who is an IV drug user has less right to treatment than a patient who developed the disease following a dental procedure?

☆ What is your reaction to patients who have contracted HIV through a blood transfusion compared to those who caught it through unprotected sex?

☆ How do you feel about smokers and their right to treatment? Do you feel they have less right to healthcare than non-smokers because they played a part in causing their health problems? Perhaps you think they have more right to treatment because they pay more towards their health insurance or to the NHS through tax on their tobacco. If so, are you saying that healthcare should be delivered according to how much you pay for it, not on how badly you need it?

☆ What do you think about people who do other risky activities, e.g. rock climbing or skiing? What about the self-employed worker who has an MI due to a stressful lifestyle?

The GMC states that doctors must 'not deny or delay investigation or treatment' of a patient who may have contributed to their condition through their actions or lifestyle. (GMC, *Serious Communicable Diseases*, Oct 1997).

Serious communicable diseases

The GMC defines a serious communicable disease as "one that may be transmitted between humans and which may result in death or serious illness" (GMC, *Serious Communicable Diseases*, Oct 1997). Examples include HIV, TB, Hepatitis B and C.

Patients

Of course, universal precautions should be used with all patients but how can you further reduce the risks to yourself and others if you know a patient has such a disease? Think about infection control measures such as double-gloving, never re-sheathing needles, wearing a mask, and using 'high-risk' stickers for specimens.

☆ Would you be happy to perform an elective operation on someone who was HIV positive? If you would be reluctant to do so, would you agree to perform emergency surgery if you were on-call?

If you are exposed to infectious material but do not know whether the patient is carrying a disease you can try to gain the patient's consent to test them. If the patient refuses, or is unable, to give consent, e.g. if unconscious, things become difficult. The GMC advice (GMC, *Serious Communicable Diseases*, Oct 1997) is that in 'exceptional circumstances' you may test a blood sample that has already been taken, but you may not take a new blood sample expressly to test for the disease. Consult your occupational health consultant and be sure you know your hospital protocol on what to do if you are exposed to infectious material.

☆ Do you think all patients should be tested for HIV or other communicable diseases? Why are they not?

Doctors

Doctors have special obligations for serious communicable diseases. The GMC states (GMC, *Serious Communicable Diseases,* Oct 1997) that if you believe a doctor has such a disease and 'is practising, or has practised, in a way which places patients at risk', the occupational health consultant must be informed or, if necessary, the GMC. Of course, it is best if the infected colleague passes on the information themselves.

Doctors with serious communicable diseases are not prevented from practising medicine altogether. Work activities will only be restricted so that patients are not placed at risk, e.g. such doctors may not carry out invasive procedures. Medical students, however, are not permitted to register with the GMC if they are known to be infected. Is this fair?

☆ Should all doctors be tested for serious communicable diseases? If the GMC has a strict policy on this, why is testing of all doctors not enforced? On what ethical grounds could you reason both sides of this argument?

☆ The GMC advises (GMC, *Serious Communicable Diseases,* Oct 1997) that you should not withhold any investigation or treatment of a patient because they are carrying a serious communicable disease. However doctors who are carriers of such diseases are not allowed to do procedures that may expose their patients to the same risks. Is this fair?

Consider that doctors (whether they are carrying a serious communicable disease or not) do not need to do invasive procedures on others to maintain their own health. Patients on the other hand may need to be treated to survive.

Stealing from the hospital

☆ How do you feel about the fact that the colleague is stealing diamorphine from the hospital? Is stealing from the hospital morally the same as stealing from a different source?

☆ Is stealing ever morally excusable? If so, does it depend on the monetary value of the object, i.e. is stealing a few paracetamol tablets for a headache better than taking a stethoscope? What would be the effect on the hospital if every member of staff were able to take as many paracetamol tablets as they wanted?

Breaking the law

Since 1 July 2002, all NHS employees have been subject to pre-appointment checks. These checks have been introduced by the Government to tighten up patient safety, as a result of various recent cases including that of Dr Harold

Shipman who was convicted of the murders of over 200 of his patients. Doctors must now let their (future) employers know if they have ever:

- been charged or convicted of a criminal offence in the UK or abroad (excluding parking tickets)
- received a police caution, final warning or reprimand.

Doctors are exempt from the Rehabilitation of Offenders Act 1974. This means that while other members of the public are allowed to withhold information relating to certain criminal offences which occurred many years ago, doctors must declare all such details no matter how long ago the incident occurred.

In addition doctors must notify their employer if they have ever been investigated for fitness to practise issues in the UK or abroad.

Finally, those doctors who may have to treat people under 18 years old are required to state whether they have ever been investigated by the police, or been dismissed from any previous employment for reasons of misconduct.

Employers have a duty to respect confidentiality and act according to the Data Protection Act 1998 when carrying out these background checks. Employers are not prevented from employing doctors who declare that they have been in trouble with the law before, but they would probably not employ someone who lied about any past convictions.

☆ Do you agree that background checks should be done on all doctors? Do you think these checks are an infringement of personal liberties or a necessary precaution?

The GMC should also be informed if a doctor is convicted of a crime. Depending on the offence, it could be regarded as serious professional misconduct with the ultimate penalty of being struck off the medical register.

Case 7 Summary

- Doctors have a duty to protect patients if they suspect that they themselves or a colleague poses a risk to the welfare of patients, e.g. is incompetent due to drug abuse, or carries a serious communicable disease.
- Doctors must inform their employers and the GMC if they have ever committed certain offences, or been investigated for fitness to practice issues.
- Patients should receive treatment for their condition regardless of how much they contributed to their ill health.

CASE 8: DEATH OF A CHILD

Issues

Post-mortem examinations
Death certificates

You are an SpR in paediatric A&E when a six-month-old baby is brought in by ambulance in severe cardiovascular shock. The baby has suffered a respiratory arrest and despite everything the hospital team does for her, she dies a few hours later. You ask the parents if you can perform a post-mortem on their child to help discover why she died. The parents are naturally distraught and are vehemently opposed to their baby "being cut up by you butchers – can't you leave us to bury her in peace?"

- **How do you deal with the situation?**
- **Should you always ask relatives for consent to post-mortems?**

Use this space to note down your own ideas…

Post-mortem examinations

There are certain situations when it may be necessary to inform the Coroner (in England or Wales) or the Procurator Fiscal (in Scotland) that a death has occurred. The exact circumstances vary but generally include any sudden, suspicious, accidental, unexpected or unexplained death. Examples include:

- any death in custody
- deaths of foster children
- suicide
- hospital-related matters.

It is then up to the Coroner or Procurator Fiscal to decide whether to investigate the death by holding an inquest and/or a post-mortem on the body. The family cannot prevent a post-mortem from going ahead if the Coroner/Procurator Fiscal has requested one to be carried out. It is therefore inappropriate to ask for consent for a post-mortem in these situations. However, it is good practice to inform them that it may be necessary.

Other occasions when a post-mortem may be indicated are when it would be of benefit to research or clinical practice. In these situations the family should be consulted and asked to consent.

Ever since it emerged in the 1990's that organs and tissues were being retained by certain hospitals without the consent of relatives, gaining consent to this practice has become a great deal more explicit.

☆ What do you think about how dead bodies should be treated? How do you treat dead bodies, e.g. during anatomy dissection sessions?

☆ Is it right that relatives can object to a post-mortem even if it may further knowledge and research into diseases and prevent future deaths occurring? Should they also be allowed to object to post-mortems ordered by the Coroner, where the sole benefit will be to establish the cause of death of one individual?

☆ Why is it important for relatives to be able to play a role in deciding the fate of another's dead body? In whose interests are we acting by maintaining this role?

☆ Does it make a difference whether a piece of tissue is kept on a slide in a hospital or buried with the rest of the body?

Death certificates

Death certificates can be issued by any doctor who attended the patient during their 'last illness' and has also seen the body after death.

If you are going to complete the death certificate for a patient you must be able to make a statement as to the cause of death. If you are unsure about why the patient died, you are under no obligation to complete the certificate and should speak to a senior about this.

On the certificate, the actual cause of death is divided into Part I and Part II. Part I should be completed with the disease or condition which directly led to death, e.g. coronary artery disease. The more specific you can be the better since mortality statistics will then be more accurate. Part II relates to other significant conditions that contributed to, but were not directly related to, the cause of death, e.g. diabetes mellitus.

A common mistake is to fill in the certificate with information that would mean the death should be reported to the coroner. Matters such as 'fractured femur', 'alcoholic cirrhosis' or 'drug overdose' will be rejected by the Registrar unless the Coroner has been notified.

Do not complete a cremation form until a death certificate has been issued.

Case 8 Summary

- If you are unsure about the cause of death, speak to a senior before completing the death certificate.
- Do not complete a cremation form until the death certificate has been issued.
- If the death is notified to the Coroner/Procurator Fiscal, the next of kin should be informed that a post-mortem may be necessary – relatives cannot prevent it from taking place.
- If a post-mortem is desired for other reasons (e.g. research), relatives must first give their consent and be told accurate information about exactly what will happen to all parts of the body including organs and tissues.

CASE 9: ORGAN DONATION

Issues

Organ donation and transplantation
Respecting cultural and religious beliefs

You are an SHO in A&E when a previously fit and well 21-year-old British Asian female is admitted following a fall from a horse. Her GCS is 10 on admission but steadily worsens and she becomes comatose. You have found an organ donor card in her pocket but when you broach the subject with her parents, they are opposed to this since it is against their religion.

- **How do you deal with this?**
- **Whose wishes should you respect?**

Use this space to note down your own ideas...

Organ donation and transplantation

Under the Human Tissue Act 1961, people who wish to donate their organs after their death can join an organ donation register and carry a donor card to indicate their wishes. Unfortunately these are not binding in law and therefore organ donation does not happen as often or as easily as it should.

In practice, if the relatives are opposed to organ donation it is **their** wishes that are respected more often than those of the deceased.

☆ Why does this happen?

☆ Is it ethical for us to go against the wishes of someone who wanted their organs to be used after their death?

A person has no legal right to determine what should happen to their body after their death. It is normally the responsibility of the next of kin, as those 'in lawful possession' of the body, to make decisions as they see appropriate.

The Code of Practice for Organ Transplantation Surgery has been in use since 1979. Its recommendations make clear that before organs are removed, death should be certified by at least two doctors (one of whom must have been qualified for at least five years; neither should be a member of the transplant team to avoid any potential conflict of interest). The Code confirms that if relatives are against the procedure their wishes should be followed, even if the deceased wished to donate their organs.

The situation for donor organs in this country is desperate. At present we have an 'opt-in' policy, where it is assumed that people do not wish their organs to be used after their death unless they have explicitly requested it. However, if we had an 'opt-out' policy where the situation was reversed and people were effectively required to carry 'non-donor cards', the number of organs available would probably increase substantially. An 'opt-out' system now exists in other countries (e.g. Austria, Belgium, Denmark, France) however some surgeons are still unwilling to remove organs without the consent of the next of kin.

☆ What are the arguments for maintaining the current 'opt-in' system for organ donation rather than an 'opt-out' policy?

☆ People are allowed to donate blood and semen while they are alive. Is there any difference between this and donating a kidney?

The Human Organ and Transplants Act 1989 allows live organ donation to occur between people who are 'genetically related' (grandparents and grandchildren are **excluded**). If a person wishes to be a live organ donor for a 'genetically unrelated person', the case must first be approved by the Unrelated Live Transplant Regulatory Authority (ULTRA). Under ULTRA regulations, incompetent persons (adult or child) cannot be live donors because they are regarded as incapable of sufficient understanding to give explicit informed consent. The GMC gives specific advice on this issue too (GMC, *Transplantation of organs from live donors*, Nov 1992).

The Human Organ and Transplants Act 1989 makes it illegal for any 'organ' to be bought or sold, whether the donor is alive or dead. Presumably ULTRA was created to ensure that non-altruistic donations never take place and to protect donors from coercion. However, although perhaps a **financial** incentive would not exist between genetically related people, there is surely an element of **emotional** coercion that would exist between family members, e.g. a brother may be put under pressure from his relatives to donate a kidney to his sister.

Under the Act, an 'organ' is defined as "... any part of a human body consisting of structured arrangement of tissues which, if wholly removed, cannot be replaced by the human body." Therefore blood and bone marrow are exempt from the Act.

The live donation of gametes (semen and ova) is covered by The Human Fertilisation and Embryology Act 1990 and regulated by the Human Fertilisation and Embryology Authority (HEFA). Under the Act, it is prohibited for live donors to be paid for their gametes unless it has been approved by HEFA. In practice, sperm donors are paid routinely whereas egg donors are rarely offered any financial incentive – yet carry the higher risk.

☆ Should sperm and egg donors be paid equally? Is there a problem with paying donors for their gametes? In France, sperm donors are not paid, and they are usually mature men who have already proved that they are capable of fathering a child. Despite this, there seems to be no shortage of willing donors so, at least in France, supply is not a problem.

☆ In some countries organs can be bought and sold on the black market. It is most often poor people who decide to sell a kidney of their own so that they can gain a substantial sum of money. Do you think this is ethical? They are undoubtedly taking a risk with their own health by doing this, and if their other kidney failed at some time in the future their health would suffer and they may die. It is therefore perhaps not in someone's best interests to lose a kidney. However, the donor may judge that the health risk is worth taking since their quality of life (with money but without a kidney) may be significantly better than if they retained both kidneys but had no money. Furthermore, other people such as boxers, and racing car drivers, take substantial risks (to health and life) to earn a living, and they are not prevented from doing so. In fact, this risk is usually recognised, and they are financially rewarded accordingly. Do you see any problems with paying donors for their organs? On what ethical grounds could you argue both sides of this debate?

☆ Technology is advancing in a way that it may soon be possible to grow organs in vitro, expressly for transplantation. Do you think this is ethical?

Respecting cultural and religious beliefs

What we regard as 'ethical' is influenced by our cultural, religious, and family background, as well as our own personal experiences and the legal position of the country in which we live. It is therefore very difficult to argue that one person's set of ethics is more 'ethical' than another's.

In the present day, where most people live within a multi-cultural society it has become necessary to develop an awareness, and a tolerance, of different cultural beliefs and customs.

☆ Do you agree that individuals have a right to maintain the beliefs and traditions of their culture or their religion? Are there circumstances when this should not be permitted?

☆ Where do you draw the line between respecting someone's different cultural beliefs and condoning immoral acts? What do you think about circumcisions done on religious grounds rather than out of medical necessity (male or female)?

In this case the deceased wished her organs to be donated while her relatives refused. It does not matter that they refused on religious grounds, they could well have refused because they 'didn't like the idea'. The relatives' decision must be respected since the deceased has no right to decide what should happen to the body after death.

☆ Do you agree with this?

It is however assumed that the relatives will respect the wishes of the deceased on how the body is treated after death. It should be recommended that people who want their organs to be donated after their death make their wishes known to their family. By initiating discussions on the subject and explaining their beliefs they may be able to encourage the relatives to carry out their request, even if it goes against the personal desires of the family.

Case 9 Summary

- People can indicate that they would like to donate their organs after their death by joining the donor register and carrying a donor card. This is not a legally binding agreement and the relatives should be consulted before organs are harvested.
- Religion, culture, family, the law and personal attitudes all contribute to forming an individual's set of values or ethics.

CASE 10: CONFIDENTIALITY AND DUTY OF CARE

Issues

Consent to investigations
Duty of care
Breaching confidentiality

Richard, a 35-year-old patient, presents with a dry cough having recently returned from a four-month-long business trip to South Africa (Johannesburg). On the point of leaving the room, he says "By the way, I'm a bit concerned – I slept with a woman while away, and I'm worried I might have picked up a dose" (acquired a sexually transmitted infection).

You counsel him before taking blood for an HIV test. He returns a week later and you have to advise him that the results show him to be HIV positive. He is married with two children, and his wife is also one of your patients. He is very upset when you raise the question of discussing the results with his wife. He says "No way! Our marriage is in enough trouble as it is!" The couple are not currently sleeping together, although his wife has noticed that he's been trying to avoid any form of intimacy and wonders why.

He then threatens to sue you for breach of confidentiality if his HIV status becomes known to his wife.

- **Do you try to contact the wife?**
- **To whom is your Duty of Care?**
- **How can you deal with this situation satisfactorily?**

Use this space to note down your own ideas …

Consent to investigations

✻ You should always obtain informed consent from a patient before performing any examination or investigation. Failure to do so constitutes an assault and/or battery.

☆ To ensure that consent for a blood test is fully 'informed', what should the patient know about? Does the information they need differ for a simple 'FBC' (Full Blood Count) test from an HIV test?

The different types of consent are discussed in Case 2 and the example of blood taking was used in explaining implied consent. In the case of HIV testing, implied consent is not sufficient as they may think you wish to do a simple blood test and not know that you will be testing their blood for this disease. Explicit consent must be obtained from the patient before an HIV test can be carried out.

☆ Why do we carry out a series of blood tests, such as FBC, LFTs, U+Es, etc. without telling patients all the details of all the tests and why we are doing them? Do you think we should be doing this?

HIV tests are covered in the guidance *Duties of a Doctor* issued by the GMC (GMC, *Serious Communicable Diseases*, Oct 1997 and GMC, *Seeking Patients' Consent*, Nov 1998). Patients are offered counselling both before and after the test is done. The reasoning behind this is to help people deal with a positive result (and the associated stigma and implications for insurance) and offer advice on safe sex.

Duty of care

As a doctor, you have a duty to care for your patients. In a hospital environment, this duty begins the minute they enter the hospital. In the general practice setting, however, this duty is extended so that anyone registered with the practice is your patient, not only when they come and visit you in your surgery.

☆ What implications are there for the GP as a result of the extended duty of care? When does your duty stop?

Breaching confidentiality

In general terms, a patient's confidentiality should only be breached in exceptional circumstances which you would be prepared to justify to the GMC or a court if necessary (see Case 1). This patient does not want to inform his wife of his HIV positive status.

☆ Do you think that this patient's wife has a right to know about his HIV status, and would you go so far as to inform her of it against his wishes?

Richard's initial reaction of anger could be due to fear and denial: of illness, his own death, losing his family, infecting his wife. You could offer help and support to Richard by being prepared to act as an intermediary in whatever capacity you can. You could also arrange for him to go for counselling with his wife.

Remember that both Richard and his wife are your patients. You want to maintain Richard's trust and respect, but at the same time you need to try to protect his wife from becoming infected. You also need to be able to offer her support if she is already infected.

It may be acceptable to go against a patient's wishes and inform sexual contacts of an infection risk. In such circumstances it is important to inform the patient of your intentions before disclosing the information.

If you think that you may need to breach Richard's confidentiality, you should agree on a deadline so that he knows that if he has not told his wife by a certain date then you will tell her. It is also a good idea in this kind of situation to ask him if he would prefer you to meet his wife alone or with him present.

☆ What would happen if you did not ensure that Richard's wife became aware of his infection and the risks to herself, and she subsequently became infected with HIV?

Technically you could be liable for negligence, as it could be said that you failed in your duty of care to the wife (who is also your patient), allowing her to be exposed to further risk of contracting HIV. This emphasises the need for good documenting; recording what you have done, said, advised or recommended as a doctor.

Case 10 Summary
- Valid informed consent should be obtained from patients before commencing any examination, investigation or treatment.
- Consent from the patient must also be obtained before discussing a patient's case with third parties.
- Confidentiality should only be breached in exceptional circumstances (outlined in Case 1).

CASE 11: THE YOUNG MOTHER

Issues

MMR
Prevention v treatment
Refusing consent for minors – parental rights
Relationship of trust

You are a GP registrar. Kylie is one of your patients, and is the 15-year-old mother of a 12-month-old baby, Britney. Kylie lives at home with her parents, who help her to look after Britney.

Britney is due soon for her MMR jab (measles, mumps and rubella immunisation). You discuss this with Kylie when she visits for a routine check-up with her mother and Britney. She is completely adamant that she only wants the single jab, not the triple jab since she has heard horror stories about its side effects. You say that you understand why she is concerned but state that you feel it is in the child's best interests to have the triple jab. Kylie replies that if you won't provide the single jab she will find another doctor who will.

The next day, Kylie's mother phones you to say that she wants Britney to have the triple jab. She says that if she offers to bring the baby in for the jab, Kylie need never know that the baby received the triple rather than the single dose.

- **Does Kylie have the right to withhold the vaccine from her daughter when you feel this would not be in the child's best interests?**
- **Since Kylie is under 16 herself can she legally consent to treatment on behalf of her daughter?**
- **As Kylie is under 16, her mother can make medical decisions on her behalf if necessary. Does this mean that she should/can make decisions for Britney too?**
- **How can you deal with situations when the parent refuses to consent to treatment which you regard as medically indicated for their child?**
- **What are the legal consequences, if any, of doing as the grandmother suggests, by acting expressly against Kylie's wishes and giving Britney the triple jab?**

Use this space to note down your own ideas...

MMR

The general public is often influenced in health matters by the Press and TV. This can be good since it raises awareness of medical issues in society. However, it may also cause anxiety levels to increase when there is no reason to worry.

The MMR vaccine is thought to be safe (and is in fact probably **safer** than the single measles jab) by most medical practitioners. However, a few cases brought to the public attention via the Press have caused concern that the MMR may increase the incidence of autism in children. This is presumably at the heart of Kylie's decision to withhold the vaccine from her daughter.

Prevention versus treatment

The purpose of vaccination is ultimately to prevent children from getting a potentially dangerous disease (e.g. measles can render a child blind or deaf, and even lead to death). Vaccinating large numbers of children works because it confers the society with 'herd immunity'. This means that the disease is largely eradicated from the population so that the risk of coming into contact with the disease is very low indeed. Therefore, unvaccinated children within the population also benefit from the herd immunity because they are only at a very low risk of catching the disease anyway as it is not around much.

However, herd immunity only works if a certain percentage of the population have been immunised. If there is a large group of children who are not vaccinated then the risk increases greatly, including to those children who are vaccinated because vaccines can only reduce the chances of getting the disease and not prevent it completely.

Vaccination is a cheap and effective way of reducing the incidence of certain diseases. It is in society's interests to maintain immunisation programmes for all members of the population at risk. Vaccination is, however, not a medical treatment; it is not a cure for a disease that the child actually has. For this reason parents have the right to refuse immunisation for their child without recourse.

☆ Do you agree that vaccination is not the same as treatment?

You could say that vaccination is in the same class of intervention as a healthy diet or exercise. All are encouraged as important in preventing disease but none are mandatory. However there are other medical interventions such as warfarinising people who have atrial fibrillation, or using beta-blockers to control hypertension which are usually thought of as treatments to prevent a stroke.

✩ Where do we draw the line between prevention and treatment? Prevention is better than cure; does it matter if there is a difference between the two, when both improve health?

Choosing not to vaccinate is perhaps more complicated as it has implications for the health of others, even those who are immunised. An analogy can be seen with smoking. By not smoking you will reduce your risk of getting lung cancer significantly. However if you are around others who smoke, your risk will increase due to passive smoking. Despite this, we have not banned smoking in public buildings (although certain countries such as the US and Italy have done this). Could you envisage nurseries which only allow vaccinated children? In some areas of the US, children are not allowed to attend school until they have received certain vaccinations.

✩ Given that not vaccinating a child could increase the risk for other children, and that herd immunity only works if a large percentage of the population have been immunised, can you argue that vaccination should be enforced? What are the grounds for allowing parents the right to choose?

Fluoridation of the water supply is an example of another public health measure that has been cheap to implement, and helped to significantly reduce the incidence of dental caries (although there are some potential side effects).

✩ Can you brainstorm a list of other initiatives that have been used to control our behaviour to improve our health? Some examples include making it illegal to travel without a seat belt in cars and setting minimum ages for buying alcohol and cigarettes. Do you agree with these restrictions on personal liberty? Do you believe these measures have been successful? The Netherlands and Italy have no restrictions on buying alcohol yet have a lower incidence of alcohol-related diseases. Can you think of any other possible solutions to health problems that could be more effective than legislation, e.g. education?

Refusing consent for minors – parental rights

As Britney's mother, Kylie has parental rights and the right to decide to refuse vaccination. As she is under 16 we cannot assume her to be competent, but if she can demonstrate that she satisfies the conditions of competence (simply refusing vaccination for Britney would not allow us to regard her as incompetent) we must obey her right to choose in this situation.

If Kylie was incompetent Britney could either be made a ward of court (see Case 5), or the courts could decide to let another party, e.g. the grandparents hold parental rights. Whatever the situation, it would no doubt be important to involve Kylie in any decision-making regarding Britney. Kylie's understanding would increase with age and experience, and her capacity to consent would evolve until she was able to assume full parental control.

☆ If Kylie was judged to be incompetent, what would be the effect of barring her from being involved in all decisions regarding the care of Britney?

☆ How far do parental rights go? Do parents always have the right to refuse treatment for their children?

In 1981 there was a case which concerned a child born with Down Syndrome and duodenal atresia. The normal course of action is to perform surgery to relieve the obstruction. The parents, however, decided that they would rather the child died naturally over the course of a few days than live handicapped for several decades – they refused consent to the operation. The surgeons believed the procedure was in the child's best interests and took the case to court.

The child was made a ward of court but the judge also refused consent to treatment. The surgeons appealed against this decision and the Court of Appeal (Re B.[1981] 1 WLR 1421) authorised the operation to go ahead. In his ruling, Lord Justice Templeman recognised that the ultimate decision should be based on the evidence and opinions of both the doctors and the parents. He acknowledged that: "There may be cases ... of severe proved damage where the future is so certain and where the life of the child is so bound to be full of pain and suffering" that it would be right to allow the child to die. However, he refused "to terminate the life of a mongoloid child because she also has an intestinal complaint."

☆ What is the effect of courts deciding against the views of the parents? Can you think of any other solutions to this problem? How would you deal with parents who refused to consent to treatment on behalf of their child, even though you believe treatment to be in the best interests of the child?

Relationship of trust

☆ What would be the effect of giving Britney the MMR without Kylie knowing?

By going against Kylie's wishes you would risk shattering any relationship you have with her, and put in jeopardy any chance to help Kylie and Britney in the future.

Legally, you risk being found guilty of assault and battery, for carrying out a procedure for which you do not have parental consent. It does not matter that

Kylie agreed in principle to an injection (the single measles vaccination) nor does it matter that Britney's health is not damaged by the triple jab. Simply by knowingly injecting a substance which the parent had expressly stated they did not want injected into their child, is enough to warrant legal proceedings.

☆ Doctors are supposed to foster a relationship of trust with their patients. Why is this important?

As long as patients feel that they can trust their doctor to make good decisions, act in their best interests and be truthful with them, the more likely they are to seek medical attention when necessary. They themselves will probably be more honest too, thereby allowing the doctor to make a more accurate diagnosis and give more appropriate advice. Working together on a management plan will mean that the patient is more likely to comply with medication, therefore increasing the efficiency of the doctor's time and energy. Mutual trust within the doctor-patient relationship benefits both parties.

Case 11 Summary

- Fostering a relationship of trust with a patient is important; it will help the doctor to form a more appropriate management plan and encourage the patient to follow medical advice.
- Parents/guardians have the right to refuse consent for their child to receive certain medical treatments (e.g. routine vaccinations).
- If doctors feel that the parents/guardians are wrong to refuse consent for their child they can apply to the courts for permission to treat.
- Administering treatment without consent could be regarded as a crime (battery or assault).

CASE 12: THE ANOREXIC PATIENT

Issues

Confidentiality
Eating Disorders and the Mental Health Act
Assessment and the Mental Health Act
Treatment and the Mental Health Act
Autonomy and paternalism

You are a GP registrar, currently attached to a busy student health practice. Emma is a 19-year-old geography student in her first year at university. She temporarily registered with you soon after the start of term in order to be started on the oral contraceptive pill (OCP).

While taking her blood pressure, you noticed that she seemed abnormally thin. You mention this, and she says: "Yeah, I haven't been eating too well – I don't like the food in Hall."

Three weeks later you are called to her Hall of Residence by the Warden – she tells you that Emma has not been out of her room for three days, and her friends are all concerned about her. Emma refuses to eat anything, saying she is fine and just wants to be left alone.

- **What do you do now? Should you speak to:**
  - **Emma directly**
  - **her friends**
  - **her parents**
  - **her home GP?**

You decide to talk to Emma in her room. She says: "Why can't you just leave me alone?" and becomes distressed. You suggest that she should allow you to refer her to the local Eating Disorders Unit or come into hospital for assessment. She refuses point blank.

- **Should you force Emma to be admitted to hospital?**
- **If she is admitted, should you force Emma to eat?**

Use this space to note down your own ideas...

Confidentiality

Emma is your patient, and as such, is entitled to the same right to confidentiality as any other patient. It is always preferable to try to speak to the patient in the first instance. This is the best way in which to help you form a diagnosis and management plan. If this fails or further information/support is required you can ask the patient's consent to speak to others (e.g. parents, friends, GP, etc.). The best way in which to approach this is by suggesting a joint meeting with the patient and the other individual(s). If the patient refuses this, then you have a duty to respect their wishes. However, considering that you are unlikely to have easy access to Emma's past medical notes (because she is registered only temporarily with you), it would be reasonable for you to contact her home GP if necessary. If she happened to be incompetent, you would be justified in breaching confidentiality in her best interests.

Eating Disorders and the Mental Health Act

The Mental Health Act 1983, the Mental Health (Scotland) Act 1984 and the Mental Health (Northern Ireland) Order 1986 provide the statutory legislation dealing with mental illness in the UK. There is little difference between the acts and, for simplicity, specific reference will be confined to the 1983 Act.

Recently, a new draft Mental Health Bill for England and Wales was put out to consultation. When in due course this Bill is amended and enacted (becomes law), it will have an impact on guidance for the involuntary detention and treatment of the mentally ill. In the meantime, you can find the consultation documents at:

http://www.doh.gov.uk/mentalhealth/draftbill2002/index.htm

The Mental Health Act Commission (MHAC), (and a similar body in Scotland) regulate and provide guidance on the implementation of the Act. A good website for information on MHAC guidance is www.hyperguide.co.uk

In order to decide what action is appropriate in this case, you first have to determine whether Emma can be considered under the Act. Patients covered by the Act must have a 'mental disorder', of which there are four categories: mental illness, mental impairment, severe mental impairment and psychopathic disorder. The Act does not define 'mental illness'; note that dependence on drugs or alcohol, and sexual deviancy (e.g. paedophilia) are **not** considered 'mental disorders'.

The latest International Classification of Diseases (ICD-10) suggests that for a definite diagnosis of anorexia nervosa all the following criteria should be met:

- body weight maintained at least 15% below expected body weight
- weight loss self-induced by avoidance of fattening foods or by one or more of the following: vomiting; purging; excessive exercise; use of appetite suppressants and/or diuretics
- body image distortion with a fear of obesity
- widespread endocrine disorder involving the hypothalamic/pituitary/ gonadal axis
- if the onset is pre-pubertal, pubertal events are delayed or arrested.

ICD-10 also refers to the occurrence of depressive or obsessional symptoms, the presence of features of a personality disorder. It is also important to exclude somatic causes of weight loss in young patients, including chronic debilitating diseases, brain tumours and gastro-intestinal disorders such as Crohn's Disease or a malabsorption syndrome.

Without proper assessment, it is impossible to say whether Emma is suffering from anorexia nervosa but you have reasonable cause to believe that she may be. More acutely, you may be concerned that she has abnormal blood chemistry due to her refusal of food. This may be affecting her ability to make a rational choice (her capacity) and may compromise her competence.

Legal cases (*Riverside Health NHS Trust v Fox* [1994] 1 FLR 614 and *B v Croydon HA* [1995] 1 All ER 683) have shown that anorexia nervosa can be described as a 'mental disorder' under the Act. The question you must ask yourself is whether Emma should be admitted. If she does need to be admitted, you must then decide whether it is necessary to resort to the Mental Health Act in order to achieve this, and which Section is most appropriate.

Assessment and the Mental Health Act

It is clear that Emma needs proper assessment before an accurate diagnosis and management plan can be decided. Assuming that she does not require emergency treatment, you have several options open to you. In order of preference, these are summarised:

- **Voluntary admission**

This is always the ideal solution if possible. It may take careful negotiation and expert communication skills to achieve this and it may be worth requesting the help of a social worker (approved under the Mental Health

Act). They will have vital experience and besides, will play an essential part in sectioning the patient if this becomes necessary.

If the patient can be convinced to come into hospital voluntarily this is a very promising start to treatment. It is important that the patient trusts you as their doctor, so you should not lie to the patient or make promises that you cannot keep. Likewise, to avoid being manipulated, do not make deals about what may or may not happen as a result of the admission.

If the patient refuses to come to hospital you could decide that a compulsory admission is **not** necessary. This may help to maintain the doctor-patient relationship that could encourage the patient to voluntarily seek your help at a later stage (see Case 11).

However, the Act will allow you to admit the patient **involuntarily** if it is 'in the interests of the patient's own health or safety or with a view to the protection of other persons'. In the case of anorexic patients this would only be in an extreme situation where the patient's health was seriously threatened by food refusal.

- **Admission for assessment – Section 2**
  - **Purpose:** Assessment.
  - **Applicant:** Nearest relative or a social worker approved under the Act. The applicant must have seen the patient in the past 14 days. The applicant is responsible for taking the patient to hospital (although this can be delegated to others e.g. ambulance personnel) and, if necessary, may use force (not excessive) to achieve this.
  - **Recommendation:** Two doctors – one must be a psychiatrist (approved under the Act), and the other should preferably have 'previous knowledge' of the patient (usually the GP).
  - **Duration:** The admission can last for up to 28 days and it cannot be renewed. If an extension is required, a separate application **for treatment** (Section 3) must be made. An appeal by the patient can be made any time within the first 14 days.
- **Emergency admission for assessment – Section 4**
  - **Purpose:** Assessment. Admission under this Section should really only be as a last resort in emergency circumstances. If it **is** necessary, you should aim to get the patient seen by a suitable doctor as soon as possible so that the admission can be approved under Section 2 instead.
  - **Applicant:** Nearest relative or approved social worker. The applicant must have seen the patient in the last 24 hours.
  - **Recommendation:** One doctor – who need not be a psychiatrist, but should ideally have 'previous knowledge' of the patient.
  - **Duration:** 72 hours.

Appeals

Patients are allowed to appeal to a Mental Health Review Tribunal (MHRT) to overturn the Section order. A tribunal consists of a lawyer, a psychiatrist and a lay person, and has the power to discharge the patient. For their appeal, patients may be given legal aid and can obtain an independent medical opinion.

Treatment and the Mental Health Act

During your assessment of Emma you may determine that she requires treatment for her anorexia. In the Act, 'medical treatment' includes "nursing and also includes care, habilitation and rehabilitation under medical supervision". For anorexic patients, treatment could take the form of counselling, psychotherapy, and nutritional advice. The Eating Disorders Association in the UK (www.edauk.com) has some specific advice regarding treatment:

"… with illnesses like anorexia or bulimia nervosa, the person must themselves want to get better before help can be really effective. People with eating disorders often have mixed feelings about 'giving up' their illness. This is because their eating habits have become a way of coping with their profound emotional problems."

This is important to bear in mind when treating these patients: they may initially not want to get better, but in order to get better, they must **first** want to get better. If Emma requires treatment for her anorexia but is refusing, then it is possible to use the Act (Section 3, summarised as follows) to force her to be admitted to receive treatment. Of course every effort should be made to convince the patient to voluntarily receive treatment, since involuntary treatment is unlikely to be very effective.

- **Admission for treatment – Section 3**
  - **Purpose:** Treatment.
  - **Applicant:** Nearest Relative (NR) or an approved social worker. The NR should at least be consulted and if they object, a court order may be needed. The applicant must have seen the patient in the last 14 days.
  - **Recommendation:** Two doctors (see Section 2 Recommendation on page 102).
  - **Duration:** 6 months. Renewable for another 6 months and then for periods of a year at a time. Appeals can be made at any time in the first 6 months, and then once during each subsequent period of renewal.

However, Section 3 of the Act can **only** be used on the grounds that the patient:

"a) is suffering from mental illness, severe mental impairment, psychopathic disorder or mental impairment and his mental disorder is of a nature or degree which makes it appropriate for him to receive treatment in a mental hospital; and

b) in the case of a psychopathic disorder or mental impairment, such treatment is likely to alleviate or prevent a deterioration in his condition; and

c) it is necessary for the health and safety of the patient or of the protection of other persons that he should receive such treatment and it cannot be provided unless he is detained under this section."

☆ The Act makes explicit that it only covers the measures required to treat the mental disorder of the patient. However, what if the patient is ill, e.g. with pneumonia, yet is competent and refusing antibiotics? Anorexic patients may require feeding – is this a treatment of the mental disorder too? Can food be regarded as a medicine?

Under the Act, treatment of physical disorders (e.g. antibiotics to treat pneumonia) can only be given if it is "sufficiently connected to the treatment for the patient's mental disorder." (Mental Health Act Commission, Guidance on the treatment of anorexia nervosa under the Mental Health Act 1983, Aug 1997).

Although food is not normally regarded as a medicine, in Tony Bland's case (*Airedale NHS Trust v Bland* [1993] AC 789; see Case 2), the House of Lords ruled that feeding a patient by artificial means can constitute medical treatment. The Courts have also accepted that naso-gastric feeding can be a medical process, forming an integral part of the treatment for anorexia nervosa (*Riverside Health NHS Trust v Fox* [1994] 1 FLR 614–622). In this case of a 37–year-old woman suffering from anorexia nervosa, the Judge recognised that: "until there is steady weight gain no other treatment can be offered for the respondent's mental condition so I hold that forced feeding if needed will be medical treatment for the mental disorder."

A similar conclusion was made in *B v Croydon Health Authority* [1995] 1 All ER 683. This case concerned a woman with a psychopathic disorder. When she was held under Section 3 she refused to eat to such an extent that she eventually required tube feeding. She brought an injunction against the hospital preventing tube feeding but the Health Authority appealed. The Appeal Court ruled that tube feeding could be permitted as a form of treatment since it is a necessary precondition for the treatment of the underlying mental disorder.

Consent to treatment for patients admitted under Section 3

Under Section 63, consent is **not required** for any treatment of the mental disorder in patients who have been admitted under Section 3. However, consent should still be sought. A person who is suffering from a mental disorder is not necessarily incapable of giving consent to treatment.

However, the patient may well be entirely able to understand the proposed treatment and its consequences, yet may reject it on irrational grounds e.g. in anorexic patients, fear that the treatment will make them 'fat'. The Eating Disorders Association's UK website (www.edauk.com) includes some very powerful personal accounts by people who have experienced these conditions. In one of these accounts, a young woman describes the anorexia as having its own identity – she even called it by a name, 'Anna' – which had supplanted hers; she felt as if she was being taken over by it, and it was eroding her free will.

The Mental Health Act Commission (MHAC) "accepts that some patients with anorexia nervosa may not have the capacity to give and sustain valid consent or that their capacity to consent may be compromised." (MHAC, *Guidance on the treatment of anorexia nervosa under the Mental Health Act 1983*, Aug 1997). Therefore in such situations, Section 63 would allow forced feeding of an anorexic patient (detained under Section 3) despite them 'competently' refusing consent.

✳ So long as the intervention is directly or indirectly a form of 'treatment' for the mental disorder, it can be allowed under the Mental Health Act.

However, what about non-essential treatment that cannot possibly be part of the management of the mental disorder (e.g. a hernia repair, sterilisation)?

We have already seen in Case 2 (*Re C (Adult: Refusal of treatment)* [1994] 1 All ER 819, [1994] 1 WLR 290, [1994] FLR 31, 15 BMLR 77), that a **competent** patient (even if they have a mental disorder) has the right to refuse interventions which have nothing to do with the treatment of their mental disorder.

However, **incompetent** adult patients present a different dilemma. In one case, a 36–year-old woman (*F v West Berkshire Health Authority* [1989] 2 All ER 545, HL) with a 'mental age' of 5 was a voluntary patient in a psychiatric hospital. During her admission she began a sexual relationship with a male patient at the same hospital. Doctors were concerned that she may become pregnant and that this was not a good idea because she would be unable to care for the child. They applied to the courts for permission to sterilise the woman. The case eventually reached the House of Lords where Lord Brandon ruled:

"… a doctor can lawfully operate on, or give other treatment to, adult patients who are incapable, for one reason or another, of consenting to his doing so, provided that the operation or other treatment concerned is in the best interests of the patient."

The House of Lords suggested however that if the proposed treatment was radical and/or irreversible (e.g. sterilisation) the doctor should seek the advice of the courts before proceeding.

The term 'best interests' causes a lot of uneasiness in the courts because it can be a very subjective viewpoint. Sometimes it is not necessarily only the interests of the patient that are considered, but those of their carers or society at large.

☆ Previously in the US, some mentally handicapped people were involuntarily sterilised because it was decided that they were incapable of being parents. Arguably, there are many people who may be unfit to be parents (e.g. paedophiles, drug addicts, girls under 16 years); would it be right for these people to be denied the opportunity to have children too? In whose interests would we be acting, and is it justified?

Autonomy and paternalism

☆ Some people regard involuntary admissions to be an infringement of their human rights. They claim the right to be as thin (or fat) as they wish, and question the validity of the diagnostic labels (e.g. 'obese') imposed by the medical profession. Do you agree with them?

☆ Forcing people to be detained or receive treatment against their will 'for their own benefit' is a form of paternalism and is thought to be unethical because it denies people their autonomy. Autonomy (the right to self-rule), however, depends on the person being able to exercise this right in normal circumstances. Could a person with a mental disorder be regarded as being incapable of doing this? Does having a mental disorder mean that it may be impossible for the person to be autonomous, simply by virtue of their condition?

☆ Arguably, treatment of their mental disorder may actually restore a patient's ability to make autonomous decisions. Is a temporary 'unethical' action (sectioning the patient and removing their autonomy) acceptable if the ultimate goal (restoring their autonomy) is 'ethical'? Can you think of any situations where this may be unacceptable (e.g. killing one person to save the lives of two others)? On what ethical principles could you argue both sides: that such an action situation would be ethical, and that it would be unethical?

Case 12 Summary

- Strict criteria must be met and certain procedures must be followed in order for a patient with a mental disorder to be detained under the Mental Health Act.
- A patient with a mental disorder may be involuntarily detained for assessment and treatment (without their consent).
- Treatment of anorexic patients is most effective if they voluntarily consent to treatment and all efforts should be made to enable this.
- If a patient detained under Section 3 requires physical treatment (e.g. tube feeding in an anorexic patient), this may be delivered without the patient's consent if it is necessary and if it will ultimately help to improve their mental disorder.

CASE 13: THE SUICIDAL PATIENT

Issues

Suicide
Treatment restrictions under the Mental Health Act
Doctors with mental disorders

You are a GP registrar. Patrick, a 74-year-old patient who is himself a retired GP, presents to your afternoon surgery.

He has been receiving treatment from you for the past four months, since his wife, Joan, died. His mood does not seem to have improved since the first time you saw him. He tells you that he has been feeling suicidal for the past few days. He says he has already worked out what to do, and has taken care of his affairs. He asks you for a repeat prescription of his tricyclic anti-depressant.

- **What should you do now? Should you:**
  - **write the prescription as requested?**
  - **discuss voluntary admission to the local psychiatric unit?**
- **What would you do if he refuses admission on this basis?**
- **If involuntarily admitted, what forms of treatment for Patrick could be permissible under the Mental Health Act?**
- **Does the fact that he is a doctor make any difference to how you should manage the situation?**

Use this space to note down your own ideas...

Suicide

Someone with the medical history of this patient who has taken such steps to plan his own death is arguably at high risk of harming and/or killing themselves. In these circumstances, issuing another repeat prescription for tricyclic antidepressants could be dangerous and potentially negligent. Patrick may have not been taking the drug recently, knowing that if he stored up enough pills he could commit suicide by overdosing on them. A better solution to his request would be to acknowledge that the tri-cyclic was not working and change his prescription to a different medicine that would be safer in cases of overdose.

The Suicide Act 1961 makes it no longer illegal to commit, or attempt to commit, suicide. However, it does state that "a person who aids, abets, counsels or procures the suicide of another or an attempt by another to commit suicide" will be held liable for their actions. A person acting to deliberately kill someone would be guilty of murder; a person causing the death of another by acting recklessly or grossly negligent, without any intention to kill, could be guilty of manslaughter. It is therefore arguably possible, though unlikely, that a doctor who continued to prescribe a tri-cyclic antidepressant to a patient such as Patrick could face charges of manslaughter or assisting suicide.

☆ If a person wishes to commit suicide can it be automatically inferred that they must have a mental illness? Do competent people have a 'right to die'? (See Case 2).

☆ Notwithstanding that doctors suffer high rates of depression and suicide, given Patrick's situation, it is understandable that he may be depressed. In fact it would probably be regarded as **abnormal** if he was not depressed and instead euphoric about his current situation. Does this mean that his depression is therefore 'normal' or should it be classed as a 'mental disorder'?

Patrick requires a psychiatric referral and may warrant urgent assessment. Obviously, this is most desirable if done with the patient's consent, and every effort should be made to obtain this. However, if he is unwilling and his condition satisfies the grounds for admission under Section 2 (or Section 4) of the Act, then this is the only option available (see Case 12).

Other Sections used to involuntarily detain persons with a mental disorder who pose a risk to themselves or others

If this scenario was not set in a GP surgery but instead the patient was in another location (e.g. home, hospital ward) there are other Sections which are important to know about, which can be implemented if necessary in certain situations. Applicants are not necessary for the following Sections.

- **Section 5(2)**
  - **Purpose:** Urgent detention of an in-patient.
  - **Recommendation:** One doctor.
  - **Duration:** 72 hours.
- **Section 5(4)**
  - **Purpose:** Urgent detention of psychiatric in-patient in the absence of a doctor.
  - **Recommendation:** Registered mental nurse.
  - **Duration:** 6 hours.
- **Section 136**
  - **Purpose:** Removal to a place of safety (usually an A&E Department).
  - **Recommendation:** Police officer.
  - **Duration:** 72 hours.

If the person is refusing to leave a building (e.g. their house), a magistrate's warrant can be issued which would allow a police officer to enter the premises in order to remove the person to a place of safety (**Section 135**). This can be done on the condition that the person is suffering from a mental disorder, being ill-treated, neglected, not under proper control or is unable to care for themselves (if living alone).

Treatment restrictions under the Mental Health Act

Assuming that Patrick requires treatment for his depression yet is refusing it, he could be detained under Section 3 of the Mental Health Act (see Case 12). As has been discussed previously (Case 12), 'medical treatment' has a relatively broad definition for the purposes of the Act.

☆ Normal therapeutic measures for depression include psychotherapy, antidepressant medications and Electro-Convulsive Therapy (ECT). Is it appropriate to administer these treatments under the Act? Do you have any reservations about carrying out any of these treatments without the patient's consent? Should there be any safeguards regarding involuntary treatment?

Treatment under the Mental Health Act is subject to the limitations imposed by certain Sections: 63 (see Case 12), 57, 58, and 62.

- **Treatment requiring consent *and* a second opinion – Section 57**

Some treatments are regarded to be so potentially hazardous that someone cannot automatically be given them **even if they do consent**. These treatments are:

- any surgical operation for destroying brain tissue or for destroying the functioning of brain tissue (e.g. lobotomy)

11

- the surgical implantation of hormones for the purposes of reducing the male sex drive.

In these cases, three people appointed by the Mental Health Act Commission (MHAC) – one doctor and two others (non-doctors) – have to certify that the person concerned has given valid consent to the procedure.

Section 57 does not only apply to people detained under the Act, it applies to all patients.

● **Treatment which requires consent *or* a second opinion – Section 58**

The treatments dealt with by this Section are:

- Long-term medication for the person's mental disorder. This is defined as over three months (since the first dose) during the patient's current period of detention under the Act. In the first three months the treatment can be given without consent, and without the Section 58 requirements being necessary. The Section is renewed if the type of medication changes.
- Electro-Convulsive Therapy (ECT). This is done under general anaesthetic and involves passing an electric current through the patient's brain. This induces a type of seizure, and is thought to be beneficial in certain types of depression and other forms of mental illness.

If the patient gives valid consent to treatment then this must be documented as is routine. If the patient either refuses consent or is incapable of giving consent then a doctor appointed by the MHAC is needed to provide a second opinion before treatment can go ahead.

Once treatment has been approved a certificate is issued. Certificates must state the plan of treatment in detail. In the case of medication, the types of medication to be given and a range of doses must be documented; in the case of ECT, the number of treatments should be stated. If the plan of treatment is to be changed, fresh certificates are first required. Healthcare staff must check that any treatment they give is covered by the certificate, if it is not, they may be liable for assault.

The provisions of Section 58 do not prevent treatment being given in an mergency, as set out in Section 62 below.

Urgent Treatment – Section 62

ɔn 57 and 58 requirements do not apply where emergency treatment
ɔssary to:

ave the patient's life

- prevent a serious deterioration in the patient's condition, so long as the treatment is not irreversible
- alleviate serious suffering so long as the treatment is neither irreversible nor hazardous; or
- prevent the patient from behaving violently or being a danger to themselves or others as long as the treatment is neither irreversible nor hazardous, and represents the minimum interference necessary.

Doctors with mental disorders

If a doctor with a psychiatric condition comes to you as a patient they should be accorded the same right to confidentiality as any other patient. However, if you felt they posed a risk to patients and they continued to practise against your advice, then you should take action (see Case 7).

Case 13 Summary

- Patients judged to be at high risk of suicide may be sectioned under the Mental Health Act.
- Treatment under the Mental Health Act is subject to limitations and may require a second opinion to be sought.
- Emergency treatment may be administered without delay in certain situations.
- Doctors who pose a risk to patients due to their psychiatric condition should be advised to stop practising until they are well enough to return to work.

CASE 14: ABORTION

Issues

Truth-telling and confidentiality
Conflicting rights
The Abortion Act 1967

You are a GP working in a small rural practice. One day a 25-year-old stock-broker, Hannah, comes to see you because she thinks she may be pregnant. You do a pregnancy test that confirms her to be at least three months pregnant. She is distraught and tells you that despite the fact that she is happily married she does not want the child because she is not ready for a family. She says that she wants to continue with her career at the moment and does not want children for at least another five years. You suggest that she should discuss the matter with her husband before making such a decision. She says that she could never do that because she knows that he really wants to start a family as soon as possible. She asks you to make a referral for an abortion.

A week later, Hannah's husband Steve comes to see you because he is worried about his wife. He says that she has recently started being sick in the morning and is very tired and irritable. He asks you if she might be pregnant.

- **What do you say to him?**
- **How do you deal with Hannah's request for an abortion?**

Use this space to note down your own ideas…

Truth-telling and confidentiality

Steve has asked you a point blank question: could his wife be pregnant? Take your time to think before you answer. If Hannah had not come to see you beforehand, based on the history and the situation, you could reasonably assume that she may be pregnant. However, she could also have gastroenteritis or another medical condition. You can say this to Steve initially and observe his reaction. By doing this you are preserving Hannah's right to confidentiality, while maintaining your duty to tell the truth.

If you think quickly enough, however, you can find out some more information before you answer sensibly, even without the benefit of knowing that Hannah is pregnant. You could ask why he thinks she might be pregnant: are they trying to conceive? What method of contraception are they using – how reliable is it and how careful have they been?

Once you have asked an initial question or two Steve's answers will let you know how he stands on the issue. It would have been useful to pose similar questions to Hannah when she had come to see you. If they are not using contraception effectively there is a high risk that Hannah may become pregnant again, and come to you requesting another abortion. This undesirable situation can be avoided by counselling her (preferably together with Steve) about contraceptive methods. This contraceptive advice should be offered as standard to any woman who has an abortion. If you do not feel able to do this yourself, you should refer the couple to a family planning clinic.

Direct questions from patients are often difficult to deflect successfully but you should try not to feel pressured into responding to such questions without thinking first. One thing you must never do is lie to patients, or to others about patients. If you feel that you cannot answer a question truthfully without betraying a patient's confidence, you can simply say that you cannot discuss patient details with the person and ask them to talk to the patient themselves. This advice of course applies to situations in which you need to maintain confidentiality. See Case 1 for a discussion of situations in which you may want to breach confidentiality.

☆ What do you think about lying? Are there times when it is OK to lie? How do you define a lie? Isn't telling the truth or misleading someone as bad as actually telling a lie? Are 'fibs' or 'white lies' acceptable? Do you think it is OK for you to lie because 'everyone does it'?

☆ Why do people need to swear to tell the 'whole truth and nothing but the truth' in court instead of just saying that they will tell 'the truth'?

☆ How do you feel when you lie? Do you ever regret it later? Is it OK as long as the other person does not find out that you lied to them?

☆ How do you feel when you find out that someone has lied to you? How do you feel about that person? Are you content to be lied to as long as you don't find out?

Conflicting rights

Rights of the fetus

☆ What is your ethical standpoint on abortion? Do you feel that a fetus has a right to be born and that therefore the mother has a duty to give birth to the fetus?

☆ Why do you think the way you do about abortion? Are you influenced by your religious beliefs, your parents' beliefs, your friends' attitudes, your personal experiences, or the legal position of your country?

☆ Are there any situations in which you would consider that it is ethical to allow an abortion?

☆ Are there any situations in which you would consider that it was unethical to allow an abortion?

The Abortion Act 1967

This Act (amended in 1990) states that a termination of pregnancy may be legally carried out under the following circumstances:

- the pregnancy has not exceeded its 24th week and that the continuance of the pregnancy would involve risk, greater than if the pregnancy were terminated, of injury to the physical or mental health of the pregnant woman or any existing children of her family; or
- the termination is necessary to prevent grave permanent injury to the physical or mental health of the pregnant woman; or
- the continuance of the pregnancy would involve risk to the life of the pregnant woman, greater than if the pregnancy were terminated; or
- there is a substantial risk that if the child were born it would suffer from such physical or mental abnormalities as to be seriously handicapped.

Two registered medical doctors must be in agreement that the grounds of the Abortion Act are satisfied. Only one registered doctor is sufficient in the rare case where an abortion is 'immediately necessary' to save the woman's life or prevent her from suffering a 'grave permanent injury' to her physical or mental health.

Abortions must be notified and the doctor needs to fill in a form detailing such matters as the method used to date the pregnancy, the grounds on which the abortion was judged to be legal, the methods of diagnosis if the fetal-handicap provision was used, the method of termination, and any complications that resulted.

☆ Do you agree with the provisions of the Abortion Act?

☆ Do you see any problems in the way the Act is worded? It could be argued that in some situations an abortion could legally take place on the grounds that the fetus is female, if what the parents desire is a boy. Is this ethical?

If you disagree with abortions you can refuse to participate in an abortion under Section 4 of the Act, which allows for conscientious objection. However, if the woman's health is at risk of 'grave permanent injury' (physical or mental) or her life is in danger and 'immediate action' is required to abort the fetus, Section 4 does not apply. In these circumstances doctors must act to protect the woman's life or health, and conscientious objection is not a defence.

The GMC advises that doctors who are morally against abortions should refer the patient to another doctor who practises in accordance with the Abortion Act. Referring the woman is not regarded as 'participating' in the abortion and therefore doctors cannot refuse to do this, even if they conscientiously object to abortions.

☆ Some doctors will organise abortions for any woman who requests one within the first three months of pregnancy. This practice is defended on the grounds that there are statistics that indicate the woman's health is at greater risk if she continues with the pregnancy than if she has an abortion within the first three months. How do you feel about this?

☆ What would be the effect on healthcare if abortions were illegal? In Ireland (and Northern Ireland) termination of pregnancy is unlawful under the Offences Against the Person Act (1862). The life of the unborn fetus must be preserved even if the mother's physical health may be severely damaged. It is also an offence for doctors in Ireland to supply information to women about abortion facilities outside the country. This situation has caused women who wish to have an abortion to go to desperate lengths to have a termination. Recently, a ship equipped with surgical staff and facilities was anchored near Dublin. Irish women were able to board this ship to have an abortion.

Abortion is a very complex issue, ethically and legally. Part of the reason for this is that there is no firm agreement on when 'life' begins and therefore when a right to 'life' exists.

For example, is fertilisation of the ovum the starting point of life? Many fertilised ova fail to implant in the womb naturally yet we do not go to heroic lengths to preserve these 'lives'. Likewise, even after implantation, up to 40% naturally abort.

Perhaps life begins at a later stage, e.g. when the primitive streak forms (at 14 days), or when brain activity can be detected (at 10 – 12 weeks), or when the fetus is capable of being born alive approximately 24 weeks but this threshold is reducing with advancing technology, or at the point of birth. Some philosophers argue that a being can only be regarded as having moral rights when it can be called a 'person'; has the capacity to value its own existence. This point in development arguably takes place long after birth has actually occurred. See *The Value of Life* by John Harris for this argument.

☆ Do you believe all beings have a right to life? Are there any qualities which a human being must possess to have this right? That is, what makes it immoral to kill a human but permissible to kill an animal or a plant?

Legally, pregnancy is divided into three sections, based on time:

- From conception to implantation: Currently, although no court has been challenged on this issue, the Abortion Act only covers the period from implantation to birth. Therefore, the 'morning-after pill' and the IUD or 'coil', which primarily act to prevent implantation of the fertilised ovum in the very early stages, are not regarded as methods of abortion. The fact that these methods may also work by dislodging an implanted embryo is overlooked because in the first few days following fertilisation (during which these methods are used) it is impossible to prove whether the embryo has implanted or not. Doctors are therefore allowed to prescribe these as ordinary treatments outside the provisions of the Abortion Act.
- From implantation to 24 weeks: When abortions may be performed on all grounds of the Abortion Act.
- From 25 weeks to birth: When abortions may be performed on particular grounds of the Abortion Act.

Legally, the mother's right to life will always take precedence over the right to life of the fetus. It is only once it is born, and therefore no longer a fetus, that it is accorded the same legal right to life as any other human being.

Father's rights

The Abortion Act gives no rights to fathers; they cannot force the woman to have an abortion or deny her an abortion against her will. In fact, there is no legal obligation to even consult with fathers to hear their opinion – although this may be morally desirable in some cases. The sole gatekeepers of the Abortion Act are the doctors and the pregnant woman.

In one case in 1978 a husband tried to prevent his wife from having an abortion (*Paton v British Pregnancy Advisory Service* [1979] QB 276). The court refused his request and he took his case to the European Commission on Human Rights. He argued that the Abortion Act infringed his right to family life, and his unborn child's right to life. The Commission dismissed his claim [1980] 3 EHRR 408 on the grounds that these rights must take second place to the rights of the mother – her health and rights were more important in the circumstances.

☆ Do you agree that fathers should not have any legal rights over their unborn children?

Case 14 Summary

- Doctors should never lie to their patients, and maintain confidentiality when appropriate.
- Abortion in the UK is illegal unless covered by one of the conditions under the Abortion Act.
- Doctors who disagree with abortions on principle must refer the patient to a doctor who practises in accordance with the Abortion Act.
- Fathers have no legal right to decide whether their unborn child should be aborted or not. However, they should be involved in the decision if the mother wishes.
- There is ethical and legal debate about when 'life' begins.

CASE 15: SEXUAL ABUSE OF MINORS

Issues

Investigation of allegations
Confidentiality and privacy
Consent from minors
Children Act 1989
Child protection orders and wardship

You are a GP registrar in an inner city practice. During a consultation about another matter, David, a 19-year-old patient of yours, tells you that during an argument with his girlfriend, Sarah (18, also a patient of yours), she told him that her father had sexually abused her when she was younger.

You know the family well. Sarah's mother, Rachel (40), is currently pregnant again with her third child. She saw you recently for an ante-natal check in the practice. She told you that – after a rocky period at home, things were much better, and that her husband was taking a real interest in the family again. For example, he was helping their younger daughter Jo (aged 13) with her homework.

- **What do you say to David?**
- **Do you inform the police?**
- **Do you make contact with Rachel, Sarah or Jo?**
- **Do you try to talk to the father?**

Use this space to note down your own ideas...

Investigation of allegations

On considering this case, your immediate thoughts may turn to the safety of the younger members of this family. It is important in the first instance, however, to remember the source of this information – it is second-hand (i.e. not from Sarah herself), and it was disclosed during a time when emotions were probably running high and where details may not have been relayed accurately.

☆ How would you go about investigating your concerns?

☆ Would your attitude change if the father was:

- unemployed and living on a council estate; or
- a chartered accountant from a wealthy suburb?

If you are concerned by allegations it is important not to get involved yourself. False accusations of child abuse can be destroying to families as well as individuals. It is important that you always discuss cases such as this with a senior. It should be your consultant or GP trainer who raises the alarm, not you as a junior member of the team.

Confidentiality and privacy

Doctors have a duty to respect the patient's confidentiality. Investigation of this case will lead to an invasion of privacy. If you considered it necessary to make contact with the family, you would have to give careful thought as to how this could be done without causing offence, which may lead to their refusal to co-operate.

There are certain situations in which confidentiality may be breached and information disclosed without the patient's permission (see Case 1).

☆ With the above information, do you think you would be able to disclose the information that you have about the family?

Consent from minors

This topic is covered in detail in Case 5.

✳ Under the law in England and Wales, children who are 'Gillick competent' can consent to treatment, but they cannot refuse it. Those who are not considered to be 'Gillick Competent' require parental consent to treatment. In these cases it is still considered good practice to involve the child as far as possible in any decision-making processes.

It is possible for a 13-year-old child to have considerable insight into a situation if they are being abused. They may, however, be too afraid to admit abuse, especially if they have been threatened.

☆ How would you go about talking to a child if you suspect that they may be being sexually abused?

The Children Act 1989

This Act of Parliament exists to protect the welfare of children. It outlines parental responsibility and guardianship as well as the mechanisms in place for the care and supervision of children whose welfare is considered to be under threat.

Child protection teams are multidisciplinary teams led by social workers brought in to investigate claims of child abuse. They also involve doctors, nurses and police officers.

Children who are under surveillance due to alleged or confirmed abuse are put on the 'At Risk Register'. As a doctor, it is possible for you to contact social services to find out if a child is on the register if you have any concerns. Some A&E departments will automatically do this whenever a child comes in. Child protection orders and wardship issues are discussed in the Children Act 1989.

Child protection orders and wardship

☆ What do you think should happen if a child's parents are unable, for any reason, to give valid consent on behalf of the minor? For example, a child of Jehovah's Witnesses may be refused a lifesaving blood transfusion by the parents. Doctors may not consider this to be in the child's best interests, and question the ability of the parents to make the decision. Are doctors, however, likely to consider the wider social consequences that may be faced if the child received blood? Perhaps the parents are taking factors such as this into consideration.

In British law there are mechanisms in place to protect minors if it is considered that their parents are not able to make unbiased decisions on their behalf.

Sometimes, if the parents are considered able to look after the child but that their judgement on a specific issue is clouded, a specific issue order may be issued. This gives the courts the ability to decide on this matter only.

Alternatively, Inherent Jurisdiction gives the High Court the power to look after anyone who is unable to look after themselves. This can take the form of an order (for example a care order, an assessment order or an emergency protection order), or it can involve making the child a 'ward of court'. This is only used in exceptional circumstances. Once a child has been made a ward of court, no decisions regarding their life can be made without consulting the courts first.

Case 15 Summary

- In English Law, children who are considered to be 'Gillick Competent' can give consent to treatment, but they cannot refuse it (see also case 5).
- The Children Act 1989 exists to protect the welfare of children.
- Courts today prefer to use Child Protection orders for specific interventions, rather than making children Wards of Court.

CASE 16: BONE MARROW TRANSPLANT AND FERTILITY TREATMENT

Issues

Fertility treatment
'Motives' for childbearing
Human Fertilisation and Embryology Act 1998
Embryo selection (designer babies)
Resource allocation and rationing

You are a GP registrar. A young couple present this afternoon in your surgery. They have one child, Jamie, four years old, who is suffering from leukaemia.

They have been trying to conceive another child for the past two years. They ask you if you will refer them for IVF treatment. They are quite open in telling you that their primary reason for wanting another child is to provide a source of likely match bone marrow for Jamie, if he needs it.

You know that your local health authority does offer IVF treatment, but that the budget has been cut this year, and there are many couples wanting it.

- **Do you refer them for IVF?**
- **Do you say anything to them about their motives for having another child?**

Use this space to note down your own ideas…

Fertility treatment

✫ What do you think about fertility treatment in general? Fertility treatment achieves what would usually happen naturally (i.e. the fertilisation of an ovum by a sperm) in situations where for some reason this does not occur. Do you find it a good thing that science enables us to help couples with difficulty conceiving, or do you hold the opinion that conception is a natural process, and if it does not happen this is part of nature and should not be tampered with?

✫ Do you know anybody who has had a child with the help of fertility treatment? Or were you or a friend born as a result of this? Have you seen couples who have had difficulty conceiving?

✫ Is there a right to have a child? Is there a duty on others to preserve such a right? Or do you think the ability to have children is a privilege?

✫ In this case, the couple already have a child. If you think that there is a right to have children, how many children does this extend to? Do they have a right to be given treatment to conceive another child?

'Motives' for childbearing

✫ People have children for different reasons. Do you think that there are 'right' and 'wrong' reasons for wanting to have a child? Would wanting to help one of your existing children be a good reason or a bad reason?

✫ How do you think the existing child would feel to know their sibling had been born in an attempt to provide 'spare parts' for them? Would they feel privileged that their parents had done everything for them; would they feel some sense of duty and obligation to the younger sibling? How might they feel if their parents didn't have another child? Would they feel that more could have been done, therefore they weren't really valued by their parents?

✫ What about the proposed child? Would they feel that they were alive simply to provide the 'spare parts'? Or would they believe that they had a very special place in the world, and that they had helped their older sibling in a way that nobody else could?

✫ If you think that motives for having children can be right or wrong, do your feelings extend to 'types' of parents? Should children be deserved? Should we stop certain people having children altogether? For example, do you think that drug abusers should be permitted to have a child? If one became pregnant, should their baby be taken into care at birth? Or should they be forced to have a termination? What about prisoners? Should they be allowed to have children? How do you feel about compulsory sterilisation of prisoners? There are examples in law of people with severe learning difficulties being sterilised because it was feared that they would not be able to look after a child (*F v West Berkshire Health Authority* [1989] 2 All ER 545 (see Case 12). Is this right?

Human Fertilisation and Embryology Act 1998

In 1984 the Government commissioned a special committee, the Warnock Committee, to look at the ethics of using human embryos. This included both fertility treatments and the use of embryos in research. It recommended that embryos be given special status in law. This was accepted by the Government, leading to the introduction of the Human Fertilisation and Embryology Act 1990. The Act of Parliament introduced the Human Fertilisation and Embryology Authority (HFEA), the Government's advisory body for any issues surrounding embryos.

Embryo selection (designer babies)

There has been a growing interest in the media about using IVF as a means of selecting embryos with certain characteristics. This may be for medical reasons. For example two parents who are carriers of cystic fibrosis may wish to select an embryo who would not have the disease. There is, however, a fear that this selection could lead to a widespread creation of 'designer babies' with specific physical attributes, intelligence and other pre-selected desirable traits.

✫ Is there anything wrong with selecting embryos for medical reasons? What about cosmetic/aesthetic reasons?

Resource allocation and rationing

This case raises the issue of resource allocation and rationing. Rationing is a very real problem in any service where funds are limited.

✫ In this situation the couple already have a child. Do you think that this should exclude them from an expensive treatment that other people with no children may also want to receive? Should their reasons for wanting the second child have any influence on your decision to refer them for a treatment that is in short supply? Consider that if these parents are successful, IVF would have created one life and saved another – is this therefore a better use of resources than giving IVF to another couple who only wish to create one life?

Case 16 Summary

- Many emotional and psychological issues are involved when children are born following fertility treatment.
- The HFEA regulates the use of stored ova and embryos.
- With advancing technology, it is now possible for people to select certain embryos for implantation. Selection could be on the basis of medical grounds, or simply due to personal preferences – although it is not currently possible to select embryos for cosmetic reasons.
- In a healthcare system with limited resources, ethical issues surrounding the allocation of funding fertility treatment are particularly complex.

CASE 17: SCARCE RESOURCES

Issues

Rationing
Allocation of resources

You are a GP principal in a rural practice concerned about your rapidly diminishing drugs budget.

A new patient, a 25-year-old male, recently diagnosed as HIV+, is going to require costly anti-retroviral treatment for the foreseeable future.

Another patient, a 55-year-old woman, whom you have known for 10 years, has just returned home following a prolonged hospital stay. She requires equally costly drug treatment for a rare heart condition.

- **What options are open to you?**
- **Does it make any difference if the heart patient is:**
  - **a nurse;**
  - **a housewife, mother and grandmother caring for her own elderly mother;**
  - **a long-term smoker, refusing to quit;**

or if the HIV patient is:

- **drug abusing and unemployed;**
- **a haemophiliac PhD scientist who has contracted HIV via infected blood products, administered while he was studying in Eastern Europe;**
- **a single parent caring for his two-year-old daughter, who contracted HIV from his former girlfriend, who has since died (she was not the mother of his daughter).**

Use this space to note down your own ideas…

Rationing

Healthcare is an expensive business. The population may never have been so healthy, never lived so long, yet still higher standards of health are sought and strived for. The fact is that improving healthcare provision is a never-ending quest and requires a bottomless pit of resources, no matter where you live or how rich your government is.

Under the current UK system there is a limit on resources available within the NHS. Rationing occurs through various mechanisms such as waiting lists, and policies on treatments (e.g. prescribing Beta-interferon to patients with multiple sclerosis) and screening programmes (e.g. the ages at which mammograms should be offered routinely to women).

☆ Most societies regard healthcare as an important and fundamental service that should be provided. In the UK, the current generation has grown up with the National Health Service and the idea that access to healthcare should be based upon need and not the ability to pay. The state funds the health service, with minimal costs borne directly by patients (though indirectly it is paid for by those who can afford to contribute through taxes). This may have helped to establish the notion that people have a 'right' to 'free' healthcare. Perhaps it is also because we feel that an adequate standard of health is so important to people's quality of life that it should be provided to everyone – anything else would be inhumane. It could be argued, however, that the standard of education or even housing that one receives has an even **greater** influence on a person's quality of life. Yet we do not allocate people to schools or houses based on their need rather than ability to pay – children with 'low IQs' are not sent to the best schools, while the most intelligent kids are left to go to the worst ones. Why should healthcare be any different?

☆ Do you think people have a right to healthcare? If so, can this right ever be forfeited, e.g. by smoking, drinking alcohol or not exercising?

Allocation of resources

Consideration of cost has become part of medical practice and training. Frequently we will choose to conduct the cheapest, rather than the best, investigation first. GPs are expected to manage their own budgets and are therefore forced to make difficult decisions that affect the care of their patients based on financial considerations.

A doctor may never have to confront the kind of dilemma presented in this case. However, the point of this case is to encourage us to think about how we make such financial decisions.

☆ Is it ethical to judge whether certain people have a greater right to healthcare based on their contribution to society or whether they are a 'nice' person?

☆ What do you do when you have two 'nice' people or two worthy types of treatment to choose between?

Some would say that doctors should not be empowered to make such judgements. They would argue that doctors are not necessarily the best people to decide on whether a particular person (or a particular treatment) is worth investing in while another is not.

However difficult and unpalatable these decisions are, someone has to make them because not everything that needs to be done can get done. The funding of the NHS and healthcare in general is a subject of constant debate and doctors have considerable power in influencing how such matters are resolved.

A study carried out in 1992 looked at the factors influencing which patients were admitted to ICU beds. It is widely assumed that such decisions are made on the basis of clinical suitability and the potential benefit of the treatment. The researchers, however, found that during the three-month period (during which nursing shortages reduced the number of beds available) "political power [in the institution], medical provincialism [one service pitted against another], and income maximisation overrode medical suitability in the provision of critical care services." (Marshall, MF et al. Influence of political power, medical provincialism and economic incentives on the rationing of surgical intensive care unit beds *Critical Care Medicine* 20 (March 1992): 387–94)

Would you be happy if a close relative of yours was denied treatment on these grounds?

☆ On what basis can rationing be done ethically?

Theories of justice

You may feel that in allocating precious resources such as healthcare to individuals within a society, it should be done fairly. However, in what way should people be treated justly and equally? Should everyone be given an equal share, or receive a share according to need, societal contribution, or merit?

There are several ethical theories of justice that could be employed. Among them are:

Utilitarian:

Striving to achieve the greatest good for the greatest number would favour public health measures e.g. vaccination, but deny expensive treatments such as heart surgery and intensive care.

Libertarian:

These theories have often influenced government policies on health services in the US. Under libertarianism, there is no **right** to healthcare, it is a **choice**. If people want healthcare they are allowed to pay for it, as with any other commodity or service: they can choose to buy as little or as much of it as they want. This benefits the rich, healthy individuals within a society but neglects the poor and the very sick. However, even in the US there is the safety net of Medicaid (for the poor) and Medicare (for the poor elderly) which are state-funded, and aim to provide a minimum standard of health service for all citizens.

Communitarian:

The counter-argument to libertarian ideas, these theories aim to distribute healthcare services according to the needs and goals of the community. How these 'needs' and 'goals' are decided upon is not defined e.g. through democracy, leaders, informed individuals.

Egalitarian:

The main aim of these theories is to ensure that everyone has an equal opportunity to succeed in life. Poor health can reduce a person's ability to achieve their goals, and therefore healthcare is provided to prevent this from happening. Beauchamp and Childress describe it as follows: "Each member of the society, irrespective of wealth or position, would have equal access to an adequate, although not maximal, level of healthcare – the exact level of access being contingent on available societal resources and public processes of decision-making."

☆ In practice, the application of some of these theories could discriminate people on the basis of gender, race or age. Old age is sometimes (though not overtly) used in some instances as a reason not to provide certain treatments, e.g. kidney dialysis. (Wing AJ. Why don't the British treat more patients with kidney failure? *British Medical Journal* 287 (1983): 1157.)

Do you agree with this? Why do you (dis)agree? Perhaps you feel that it is in society's interests to help the younger individuals because they have longer life expectancies and their lives are potentially more useful than those of older people. However, it could be argued that an older person, having worked and contributed to society for 50 years (and even perhaps fought in a World War), **deserves** at least the same right to healthcare as younger members of the society.

The concept of quality-adjusted life-years (QALYs) is an attempt to reconcile the two goals of quantity and quality of life. The aim is to maximise both through health policies. In 1989 the US state of Oregon made policies regarding the state funding of healthcare based primarily on estimates of net benefits to quality of life. Committees ranked the importance of various aspects of healthcare, and therefore how much money should be spent on each area. Certain types of care, such as that of extremely premature babies, were low on the priority list because there was minimal improvement to their quality of life.

☆ However, who can judge the quality of another's life and how much a person **values** being alive? There are people who would hate to live if they lost a leg, yet there are wheelchair-bound people who would value their lives just as much as if they lost both legs. Everyone has different thresholds and values life for different reasons. Is it possible to make ethical judgements about another person's quality of life?

Some philosophers argue that it is impossible to choose between people. One potential solution is to have a form of lottery to distribute healthcare services.

For a more complete examination of the ethics involved in resource distribution see Chapter 5 of John Harris's book *The Value of Life*.

Case 17 Summary

- Rationing of healthcare resources is necessary in most societies.
- Management plans and treatment options are affected by economic considerations.
- Doctors have influence on how decisions and funding policies are made.
- There are different ethical theories on the best way to achieve justice through the rationing process.

CASE 18: RELATIONSHIPS WITH PATIENTS

Issues

Personal relationships with patients
Professional responsibilities of medical students

You are a heterosexual female final year medical student currently attached to a medical firm. You have got to know John, a 21-year-old patient, over the past fortnight. You clerked him in on admission, know his medical history, and have examined him during the course of this time.

Additionally, you have chatted with him each day, and have taken an interest in his recovery. Today, as he is packing his bag to go home, he gives you a 'thank you' card, and asks if you would "like to go for a drink sometime?"

- **John is attractive and you have lots in common. Do you agree to go out on a date with him?**
- **If 'John' was in fact 'Jane' and she suggested you meet up for a 'friendly' night out, would you go?**

Use this space to note down your own ideas...

Personal relationships with patients

✭ Would you feel comfortable going on a date with a patient? Do you think this situation is in any way similar to a middle-aged patient inviting you round to dinner at their house 'if you feel like getting away from it all and having some home-cooked food'? If not, would this second situation be acceptable?

The GMC gives guidance in *Good Medical Practice*, stating that 'In particular, you must not use your professional position to establish or pursue a sexual or improper emotional relationship with a patient or someone close to them.' (GMC, *Good Medical Practice*, May 2001).

✭ What do you think is meant by 'improper emotional relationship'? Do you think that there is any other group of people you come across in your work, other than your patients, with whom it would not be appropriate to go on a date?

Professional responsibilities of medical students

As a medical student, the GMC expects you to adopt the same professional standards as doctors and structures the curriculum for medical schools in terms of knowledge, skills and attitudes (GMC, *Tomorrow's Doctors,* July 2002). You are expected to develop professional attitudes while studying.

Case 18 Summary
- GMC guidance advises that you must not use your position as a doctor to establish emotional relationships with your patients.
- Medical students are encouraged to develop professional attitudes and follow guidance appropriate to registered doctors.

CASE 19: PERFORMING INTIMATE EXAMINATIONS

Issues

Investigation of allegations and rumours
Obtaining consent for examinations
Students in operating theatres as assistants
Patients who lack competence
Liability when no consent is obtained
Admission of errors to patients and apologies

Part 1

You are the clinical dean of your medical school. Last night at a social event, you heard on the medical grapevine that one of your consultant surgical colleagues in a nearby teaching hospital is bullying third year students into carrying out intimate examinations of patients under general anaesthetic. These examinations have not been consented to by the patients.

One of your students comes to see you this morning, and bursts into tears as she tells you a similar story. She is deeply upset about it, and feels guilty. She is talking about tracking down the patient to apologise personally for (in her words) "assaulting her like that".

- **What should you say to the student?**
- **How do you deal with the situation:**
  - **Do you investigate?**
  - **Inform others in the Faculty?**
  - **Inform the GMC?**

Use this space to note down your own ideas...

This case raises a topical issue in the area of medical education. Historically, medical students were often taught by methods which 'used' patients as 'subjects'. Patients didn't always know what was happening, partly because 'what they didn't know wouldn't hurt them'.

Ways of thinking have changed. Patients now expect to be involved in their care, and as part of this they want to know how and when they can help the training of future doctors. Many patients are delighted to help. However they want to be informed of what is happening to them.

Investigation of allegations and rumours

Hospitals and medical schools are close 'communities'. Rumours develop and circulate around such communities with amazing frequency. The question is, when do you ignore a rumour, when do you pass it on to your friends, and when do you think 'this doesn't sound right, I'd better do something about this'?

The answer to these questions will probably depend on the circumstances, and on the details of the rumour.

✫ What would you do if you heard a rumour about a friend or colleague?

A new Act of Parliament came into force in 1998 called the 'Public Interest Disclosure Act' (but commonly known as the 'Whistle Blowing Act'). This was designed to protect employees by protecting anybody who 'blew the whistle' (informed the authorities) on a colleague from being victimised or dismissed.

Obtaining consent for examinations

Did you know that it is illegal to 'touch' a person without their consent? Doing so constitutes an act of assault. There are exceptions to this in medicine, such as when a patient is brought unconscious into an emergency department and they are unable to give consent, but as a general rule you **must** obtain consent before you examine anybody.

Consent does not necessarily need to be written down. A patient can imply that they give consent – for example when you want to take blood from them. By offering you their arm with their sleeve rolled up the patient is effectively saying: "I am happy for you to do this". Consent can also be given verbally by a patient.

In practice, doctors tend to formalise the procedure of obtaining consent by asking patients to sign a form. Although this is legally no better than a verbal agreement, it lends weight to the process, ensures that it has been done and provides evidence if necessary.

☆ What do you need to do to obtain valid consent from a patient for an examination or procedure?

✳ Consent must be given by a competent individual (see Case 2) and should be both voluntary and informed in order to be valid.

The Department of Health (*Reference Guide to Consent for Examination or Treatment*, Department of Health, March 2001) has issued guidelines about obtaining consent, which state that ideally the person who will perform the procedure should obtain consent from the patient. Because this is not always possible in a busy hospital environment, doctors can delegate this task to somebody who is

- trained; and
- understands the procedure including its possible side-effects and complications.

Advice for obtaining informed consent

As a junior doctor, particularly in surgery, you will be required to obtain informed consent from patients. The GMC gives advice on this in *Seeking Patients' Consent* (Nov 1998). When doing this you should make the patient aware of the following:

- why the procedure is being proposed and the alternatives (including the option not to treat)
- what will happen during the procedure
- whether it will take place under sedation or local/general anaesthetic
- of significant risks and complications (i.e. risks that are significant in the percentage of patients they affect (e.g. pain is a common problem), or in their nature (e.g. impotence, death))
- of proposed pre-procedure requirements (e.g. fasting) and post-procedure care (e.g. bed rest, catheters, drains, etc.)
- of prognosis including possible outcomes, findings and diagnoses
- that it may not be you who does the procedure
- that anything unnecessary will not be done
- that anything necessary will be done unless they specifically say that there is something they do not want to be done
- that they may ask any questions at any time
- that they may change their mind at any time
- the extent to which students or doctors in training may be involved in the procedure

Intimate examinations

What is an 'intimate' examination? You may believe that all examinations are intimate, as they involve an individual allowing their doctor (or a student) to touch them.

Certain examinations require added respect, as they involve a greater invasion of the patient's personal space. These examinations include those of the rectum, groin, breast, internal examinations in women and examinations of the male genitalia.

☆ What is different about performing an intimate examination, compared with any other examination?

To perform an intimate examination you need to go through the same procedure of obtaining consent as you would for any other examination of a person. The fact that you may find it a slightly embarrassing subject to talk about does not exclude you from asking the patient's permission.

☆ What can you think of that a patient may want to know before giving their consent for you to perform a procedure?

In the case of an intimate examination, you may want to ensure that the following points have been emphasised:

- you are a medical student
- you are the student who will be doing the examination
- you will be doing it as an educational exercise
- you will be supervised by a qualified member of staff
- the examination will also be performed for diagnostic purposes by a doctor
- they do not have to give consent, and that if they would prefer not to be involved their own medical care will not be affected

Examinations under anaesthetic

You may be given the opportunity to perform intimate examinations on patients while they are anaesthetised for an operation. Some people consider this to be a valuable experience as it allows students to become confident at recognising 'normal' as well as 'abnormal', while at the same time removing any possible embarrassment or unnecessary pain for the patient.

Such examinations are not exempted from the need to obtain consent from the patient. In fact, the very nature of the examination coupled with the patient's lack of awareness at the time of the event makes it all the more important that you ask permission when the patient is awake, and preferably when they haven't got far more important things to worry about!

Students in operating theatres as assistants

Assisting an operation can be a very enjoyable and valuable learning experience for junior doctors and medical students.

☆ Usually an assistant in theatre would examine the area of the body that is being operated upon. This may involve performing an intimate examination. If you are a student and you are asked to do this, what should you do about obtaining consent? Or is this just part of the job of the assistant? What do you think?

This is a question asked by many, and it is a difficult one to answer. Strictly speaking, as a student, doctors should not depend on your examination findings. They should therefore repeat any examination that you perform to confirm the findings. This essentially means that anything you do is being done for your own educational purposes and not for the benefit of the patient.

If this is the case then you must obtain consent for any examinations you perform on a patient.

Regarding assisting operations in general, it is good practice to meet the patient before you perform any surgery on them. Doctors (surgeons and anaesthetists) introduce themselves to their patients, so why shouldn't you as a student? If you spend some time chatting to them before their op they will often ask if you'll be watching. Even if they don't ask, you can always say to them 'As long as it's OK with you I'll be watching the op, and I'll pop back to say hi when you come round afterwards'. A discussion such as this can easily be extended to discuss assisting the surgeon.

A patient approached in this manner is usually delighted to help (and actually glad to know someone will be watching who can come and tell them all the juicy details about how it went afterwards!)

Patients who lack competence

✳ What do you remember about assessing a patient's competence? (See Cases 2 and 5)

☆ How should you best treat a patient who is not competent to give consent to a procedure?

You may be able to think of situations where patients are not competent (for example, after an accident), but where you really need to treat them now if they are to have any chance of survival.

It is possible for doctors to treat without consent in situations like this, as long as the treatment is deemed to be in the best interests of the patient (*F v West Berkshire HA* [1989] All ER 545).

☆ Under what circumstances (if any) do you think it is acceptable for a medical student to perform a physical examination on a patient who lacks competence to give consent? What about an intimate examination?

Liability where no consent is obtained

Matters such as these have not been tested in the courts in the UK, so the following points are purely speculative.

If a person performs an act without first having obtained valid informed consent they risk facing criminal prosecution for assault and/or a civil action (trespassers to the person or negligence). They could be held personally liable. However in the case of an NHS employee, the trust for which the individual worked could also be held 'vicariously' liable. (In the case of medical students the university and medical school could be vicariously liable.)

Medical students are not solely responsible for their actions. If they are instructed to carry out a procedure by a doctor, the doctor has some responsibility for the outcomes that arise. This means that if you perform an examination without consent, the doctor who supervises you is also liable to charges of assault.

As well as the issue of assault, there is a chance of supervising doctors being held negligent following cases of examinations on anaesthetised patients. A patient under anaesthetic is (albeit temporarily) incompetent to give consent.

✳ When a patient is not competent, the role of the doctor is to administer medical treatment that is considered necessary and in the best interests of the patient.

☆ Can you think of any situations where an educational examination by a student on a patient who has not given consent, is in the best interests of that patient?

A doctor who does not act in the best interests of an incompetent patient may be found negligent.

Admission of errors to patients

The student concerned in this case considered informing the patient of what had happened.

☆ What would you do if you were placed in a similar position? Would you inform the patient? What would you tell them?

Defence organisations agree that if doctors showed empathy towards patients' complaints and apologised for mistakes, the amount of litigation against the medical profession would drop significantly. Apologising to a patient may make them feel better and may not necessarily be an admission of guilt on your part. Even simple apologies such as: "I'm sorry you have had to wait so long," or "I'm sorry that you feel you have not been well looked after," can go a long way to helping patients feel that they have been listened to and therefore reduce the likelihood that they will put in a complaint.

Part 2

Two weeks later another woman patient finds out that an illegal intimate examination has been performed on her during an exploratory operation, this time by two male medical students, and under the direction of the same surgical consultant.

One of the operating department practitioners was a neighbour of the patient, and was shocked to see her examined without any apparent consent. The Operating Department Practitioner (ODP) told the woman what had happened, including the fact that the consultant had threatened the students with expulsion from his firm if they failed to examine the woman as demanded of them.

Think about this one yourself, and try to consider what action you may have taken if you had been the ODP.

- **Should it make any difference if the patient is your friend or relative?**
- **Would you have spoken up in the operating theatre in defence of the students?**
- **How might you go about raising concerns in a situation such as this?**

Case 19 Summary

- Performing any examination without consent could result in criminal prosecution for assault or a civil action.
- Obtaining informed consent is an in-depth procedure, which involves giving information about what you are going to do, and of any risks involved.
- Examinations carried out by students, and those done when patients are under anaesthetic must be done with consent, just like any other examination.
- Apologising to patients is not the same as admitting responsibility, and is recommended by defence organisations as an appropriate action following mistakes.

CASE 20: CHEATING IN EXAMS

Issues

Cheating and plagiarism
Investigation of alleged poor conduct
Reporting concerns about colleagues

You are a medical SHO. You are on night duty when you get a phone call from an old friend from medical school who has just found out that she failed the recent MRCP exam. She alleges that one of the examiners (a recently appointed consultant in your hospital) met her on a course two weeks before the exam and offered to help her get through if "she was nice to him". She claims to have rejected his advances, but was too embarrassed to make a formal complaint to anyone. She is obviously upset and asks your advice. You are due to start working for this consultant next month as part of your rotation.

- **Do you believe her?**
- **Do you suggest she contacts:**
  - **the BMA?**
  - **the Royal College of Physicians?**
  - **the GMC?**
  - **her mum?**
- **Do you try to find another job to avoid working with the consultant in question?**

Use this space to note down your own ideas...

Cheating and plagiarism

☆ What do you think about cheats? What about doctors who cheat? Do you think it's incompatible for doctors to be cheats, or can they cheat in exams and still be good doctors?

Research has shown that many medical students do cheat, in one form or another (Rennie SC, Crosby JR *Are 'tomorrow's doctors' honest?* Questionnaire study exploring medical students' attitudes and reported behaviour on academic misconduct, *British Medical Journal* 2001; 322: 274–275). People have different ideas about what constitutes cheating.

☆ Think about the following. Do you think that they are forms of cheating?

- Forging your absent friend's signature on an attendance register, or forging your consultant's signature in a personal log of procedures you have performed
- Copying your SSM from that of a friend at a different medical school
- Copying an elective report from the Internet
- Writing in the notes 'chest clear, respiratory rate 16, trachea central' but not actually performing an examination at all.

☆ Have you ever cheated? How did you feel about doing it? What were the consequences? What do you think would have happened if you had been found out?

People fool themselves into thinking that plagiarism is not cheating. Plagiarism is a form of cheating and is always regarded as a serious offence. It can be avoided by ensuring that you reference all your work according to the guidelines laid out by your medical school/journal.

Investigation of alleged poor conduct

☆ We have already discussed the issue of what you would do if you heard a rumour about somebody. Would you ignore it or would you find out more and possibly inform somebody in an authoritative position?

☆ What action would you want to have taken if rumours were floating around about you?

☆ What would be the consequences for you, both as a doctor and the consultant's colleague, if you did inform somebody? What if you didn't?

Reporting concerns about colleagues

☆ Does it matter that you will soon be working for this consultant? Should this have any bearing on your decision to report your concerns?

☆ This consultant may be well known among his peers as someone who is of dubious character. Would you want to be associated with him if he was behaving unprofessionally? If you did associate with him, what do you think your other colleagues would think of you?

☆ How would you go about reporting your concerns?

The Public Interest Disclosure Act ('Whistle Blowing Act' – see Cases 6 and 19) was established to make informing on poor conduct of work colleagues much easier.

Case 20 Summary

- Rumours often float around hospitals. Taking action on a rumour should be done cautiously; in the first instance, aiming to ensure that it is true.

CHAPTER 5: ETHICS AND LAW IN PRACTICE

PRACTICAL ETHICS AND LAW AROUND THE WORLD

In this chapter we present a range of cases from around the world, which describe the kind of ethical and legal dilemmas that have been encountered by doctors at all levels of training and in different specialities. The cases describe real scenarios, however, patient data has been altered to ensure anonymity and protect confidentiality.

The final section encourages you to see patient complaints in a positive way, and to recognise that mistakes will occur – it is how you respond after a mistake has occurred which will mark you out as a good and ethical doctor.

ETHICS AND LAW IN EMERGENCY MEDICINE

Case 1 – Professor Peter Rosen – San Diego (CA), USA

The police brought a 32-year-old man into the Emergency Department. He had a gun shot wound of the right leg that was soft tissue only and apparently contained a bullet or bullet fragment. The bone was intact and this apparently had been a ricochet injury, according to the police. The patient wasn't telling anyone how the injury had been sustained.

Their report was that the patient had sustained the injury during a robbery that he was committing. It was alleged that he had shot and killed a convenience store clerk and had been shot by a police officer but had made a successful getaway. He was under arrest for suspicion of the robbery and murder. The police had a court order for the wound to be explored, and the bullet removed as evidence. The court order mandated exploration by any physician.

On physical examination, the patient had normal vital signs. There was a soft tissue injury of the right calf that was neither infected nor extensive. A bullet fragment or bullet could not be palpated. An X-ray study of the leg revealed the bullet fragment, with intact bony structures. The issues in the case are the ethical concerns of the physician for the patient, versus the legal request of the police to help them acquire evidence to convict their suspect.

On medical grounds, there was no reason to explore the wound. Contrary to popular Hollywood tradition, there is no special need to remove bullet fragments, especially when there is no impending damage to nerve, artery or bone, and no sign of infection. The wound was actually healing nicely, and would do perfectly well with no medical interventions.

As a physician, my first ethical obligation is to the patient. It is not up to the physician to judge how the patient is injured, and there is no way I could produce a convincing argument that operating upon the leg would help this patient. There is no law that states a prisoner has to accept medical treatment, and this patient wished to refuse all medical care. So from a medical ethical point of view, there was no reason to treat the patient further. Legally there are of course constraints upon any physician. In all jurisdictions with which I am familiar in the United States, there is a legal mandate to report wounds of violence, especially gun shot wounds. That wasn't an issue here since the police were aware of the wound and had been the ones to bring the patient to the Emergency Department.

The difficult ethical issue is whether the physician has to abide by the court order. While there may be a personal wish to support society over the individual, I found it impossible to justify performing an operation upon the patient that could not be deemed helpful in any way to the patient, even though it might be easily deemed helpful to the society at large.

I therefore refused to obey the court order. It seems to me that physicians have an ethical obligation to their profession that supersedes their ethical and, at times, legal obligation to their society. I have always felt revulsion at the physicians who acquiesced to the Austrian Empress's Law that prisoners be examined to assure that they were in good enough physical condition to withstand torture. There are numerous other societies who have had physicians place the society ahead of the patient's needs, but I think this is an abandonment of the Hippocratic tradition that has stood up well for 2,000 years.

The outcome of the case was that the patient was returned to jail, and other sources of evidence were found to enable his conviction. The police were not especially happy with my refusal, and I never talked to a judge, but I still feel strongly that this is a case where the physician's duty to the patient must take precedence over his duty to society.

Professor Peter Rosen MD FACEP FACS
Professor of Clinical Medicine and Surgery and Director of Education
Department of Emergency Medicine
University of California
San Diego, (CA), USA

Case 2 – Dr Andrew Swain – Palmerston North, New Zealand

A 69-year-old man arrived by ambulance to the Emergency Department, accompanied by his family. His main complaint was of a significant haemoptysis 1–2 hours before. The history from the family indicated that the patient had been suffering from metastatic carcinoma of the lung that had spread to the liver and involved the oesophagus. He had been a long-standing heavy smoker. The patient's regular opioid medication had been administered that day. A first course of chemotherapy had just been completed.

Examination showed that the patient was severely centrally cyanosed and dyspnoeic. His respiratory rate was over 40 per minute. He was unable to answer questions and could only grunt. His oxygen saturation was only 85% on 12 litres per minute of oxygen administered through a reservoir mask. Rales were present throughout the chest. Progressively the patient's breathing fatigued and his ventilation had to be maintained with a bag-valve-mask. His blood pressure was elevated, there were no signs of cardiac failure and there was no fever. The ECG revealed sinus tachycardia only.

The prognosis was explained to the family. The daughter did not accept that death appeared imminent and she wanted all life-saving treatment to be administered. At this point, the hospital records arrived. The histology report confirmed small cell carcinoma and the specialist considered that unless there was any prompt benefit from chemotherapy, the prognosis was abysmal.

At this point, the admitting physician attended and recommended high-dose antibiotics intravenously (piperacillin and gentamicin) despite the absence of any signs of septic shock and the main complaint of haemoptysis. The physician told the relatives that 'extremely strong medication' was being given and that this was the best that medicine could offer. Opioid was withheld to avoid further respiratory compromise. The patient died from respiratory failure in the emergency department approximately 15 minutes after the antibiotics had been administered, before he could be transferred to a ward.

What issues made it difficult?

- Lack of preparation and state of denial manifested by the relatives.
- False hope, given by the physician, that intravenous antibiotics would rectify the problem when the patient was drowning in haemoptysis fluid.
- The relatives were misled.
- Misuse of expensive antibiotics without clinical justification.
- Withholding of intravenous opioid which could have made the patient more comfortable pending his almost inevitable demise.

What did I do?

I acquiesced with this management plan as the physician had moved in to take over the patient's care and had spoken to the relatives. I did not want to cause any further distress.

What did I learn from it?

- To pursue the strength of my own convictions.
- To have managed the patient myself.
- To have advised the relatives that the prognosis was extremely bleak.
- To have supported ventilation and given adequate opioid analgesia while remaining with the patient until death, to have ensured that he was as comfortable as possible in the circumstances.
- To have withheld expensive antibiotics that were engendering false hope and were given without clinical justification.

Dr Andrew Swain FRCS
Clinical Director, Emergency Department
Palmerston North Hospital
Palmerston North, New Zealand

Case 3 – Dr Sophie Frankland – London, England

A 25-year-old man is brought into A&E by ambulance at 4 am. He has 35% second and third degree burns to his face, chest and upper limbs. On arrival to the department he is alert with a Glasgow Coma Score (GCS) of 15.

The ambulance-crew report that this man was picked up from a sauna in a 'massage parlour'. The man had apparently fainted and fallen forwards onto the hot coals in the sauna. When asked if he had any family we could contact, the man stated he had no partner and did not want his parents to know his whereabouts. It soon became obvious this man required urgent intubation and had a significant risk of mortality. Before intubation, the lead nurse asked again for relatives' details which he refused. His friend arrived soon after intubation, having left the sauna before the accident. He revealed the man did in fact have a girlfriend and a one-year-old child.

Difficult issues

- This man had significant burns to his face, arms and chest, which posed a significant threat to life.
- He required intubation due to the risk of airway oedema and for safe transfer.
- He would undoubtedly have, at best, severe burn scars for life.
- Due to his serious injuries, we would under normal circumstances contact relatives. We had to transfer him to another hospital for specialist burns care and were keen to let at least his mother know. Would this then leave his mother with the task of telling his girlfriend?

- Could we reveal the man's whereabouts without alluding to the cause of his injuries?

What did I do?

- Firstly this man's clinical situation was stabilised and arrangements made for a safe and urgent transfer
- After discussion with my consultant, we asked the police to visit his mother's house and inform her that her son was very unwell and was to be transferred to a specialist hospital. The mechanism of injury was not explained.

What I learnt

- Issues surrounding consent can be very difficult, even if no clinical information is revealed other than the patient's presence in hospital.
- To allow an individual to make an informed decision, time is required to explain implications of the injury and subsequent decisions. In the emergency situation, this is not always possible and a decision thought to be in the 'patient's best interests' may be made.
- 'Value' reactions towards a patient's mechanism of injury should play no role in the clinical management of a patient, although objectivity may be very hard to practise.

Dr Sophie Elizabeth Frankland
Senior House Officer in A&E and Anatomy Demonstrator
Royal Free Hospital
London, England

ETHICS AND LAW IN GENERAL PRACTICE

Case 1 – Dr Emma Nelson – Dublin, Ireland

Ciara was 17 and attending a psychiatrist for help with anorexia nervosa. Her potassium levels had to be monitored due to a tendency for them to drop as a result of her vomiting. This, and support, were my main roles in her care as her GP. She always attended alone and phoned for her results and follow-up plan. On this occasion her potassium level was 3.2mM/L (normal range 3.5–5.0), requiring a prescription for supplements. However it was her father who phoned, demanding to know the result. He was angry and quite aggressive, stating that she was legally a minor and that as her father he had a right to know.

The challenges

- Balancing an appreciation of his obvious distress and worry, and the need to protect Ciara and my relationship with her.
- Dealing with anger in the context of an ethical dilemma and the sense of immediacy and urgency that this angry telephone contact instilled in me.
- I was relatively inexperienced at the time and conscious of not being absolutely sure where I stood 'legally', though I felt sure what was right ethically (or rather what felt right).
- I had no idea what Ciara's wishes would be in relation to me communicating with her father.

I explained the importance of confidentiality and trust, most particularly in this age group, and that I would like to give the result to Ciara directly as I had done previously. However, threatened with lawyers and the Medical Council, I finally crumbled and gave him the result and treatment needed. Luckily my relationship with her was unaffected. It turned out she had known he was calling and was unperturbed by this. It could have been very different, particularly with a condition that tends to wreak havoc in families and in teen-adult relationships generally.

I now teach Teen Health to undergraduates and to GP Registrars and always use this case to illustrate the importance of, and difficulties with, confidentiality in dealing with teenagers. Issues they invariably debate include:

- Does the previous level of involvement of the family in the illness and its care influence the management of the dilemma?
- Should a doctor be influenced by whether or not a teenager is living independently from parents?

- Does an insight into the relationship between a teenager and parents dictate in any way how such a situation is managed?
- Would the scenario be different if her potassium result had been 2.1mM/L?
- Degrees of disclosure of information to a third party; is there such a thing as breaking confidentiality 'a bit'?

It also acts as a springboard to discussing dealing with confrontation, managing the needs of concerned relatives while preserving confidentiality, and pitfalls of communicating results. Students often ask what I did and appreciate honesty in my response. This critical incident has meant that I now clarify with teenagers who require investigation, at the outset, how they would wish me to proceed should such a situation arise.

Dr Emma Nelson
General Practitioner
Lecturer in General Practice, Royal College of Surgeons, Ireland
Programme Director, NAHB & RCSI General Practice Training Programme
Dublin, Ireland

Case 2 – Dr Dhruv Mankad – Nasik, India

I was returning from a community health education session in a village, at around midnight. On the way, a middle-aged man, Raghu rushed out waving his hands to stop our vehicle.

"Doctor please see my daughter," Raghu said. Raghu's nine-year-old daughter Nanda had had high fever since the evening with vomiting and neck rigidity. Clinically, it was acute meningitis.

"Let us go to the nearest hospital," I advised. The nearest hospital was about an hour from her village. Raghu had returned from the market town by the last bus. There were no vehicles in the villages around. To my shock her father said: 'No, please take us to a witch doctor because this is black magic." I argued with him, and spoke to Nanda's mother and to the other villagers to convince the father that there was a danger to Nanda's life and if hospitalised early, she could be saved.

The community believed the nearest referral hospital with all the facilities was a death den; this was because serious cases were always referred from villages in the district, and mortality was high. The tribe, which is dominant in the area, has several cultural beliefs different from the middle class. Education was poor and female literacy was only 7%.

Nanda's parents refused and the villagers kept silent, leaving the decision to Raghu. We waited but Raghu did not budge.

The dilemma

My ethical dilemma was should I or should I not move her to the hospital without her father's consent?

Though they had an irrational belief and faith in the witch doctor, I had the utmost respect for their cultural beliefs. I needed her father's consent because she was a minor and semi-conscious. If I moved her without their consent and she died on the way, or at the hospital, my driver and I could have been accused of moving her without consent. This would be a risk with this particular community because we had only just initiated development work with them and our relationship was new. The community could also accuse her parents of not following their traditional faith. It would also have hurt their beliefs.

The people's livelihood was from single crop agriculture with some supple-mentary source of wage labour from the Government. Cost of referring is high even if the Government hospital is free, as there is the cost of prescribed medicine, and loss of wages of two people accompanying the patient. Even if moved without consent, treating her would be a costly affair, which someone would have to bear. Moving her would mean a cost equiv-alent to their three months' income. However, not moving her had the risk of delay and of death.

What happened

An hour later, we finally left her after giving her injection penicillin, and an NSAID. We returned early next morning with adequate medicines to provide her treatment even in the witch doctor's presence. We were told, however, that she had had a convulsion an hour earlier and had died. I felt sad and dejected.

What I learnt

I learned that in a life-threatening emergency, try to seek consent from the patient's relative with witnesses around. If no consent is given, do what you think is best to save her life after informing her relatives, no matter what may be the risk. In a developing country such as India, once a good rapport with the community had been established, it would have been possible for me to take Nanda to the hospital even though her parents refused to consent. I believe, however, that in developed countries with good healthcare facilities, awareness about the individual's freedom is high, and the individual's beliefs and choices vary a great deal.

This case occurred in the 1980's, and since then we have started to train local community health workers to diagnose and treat simple illnesses, and diagnose and refer early seriously ill patients. As a development organisation, we also facilitated their pre-primary and primary education. The witch doctor is no longer functioning even though there is no doctor at all except at the local Primary Health Centre and at the referral hospital where they were earlier. Morbidity at the referral hospital remains high, but the education facilities have increased and the female literacy rate has doubled.

Dr Dhruv Mankad MB BS
MacArthur Fellow working on primary health care issues in rural areas
Nasik, India

ETHICS AND LAW IN OCCUPATIONAL HEALTH

Dr Joan Saary – Toronto, Canada

The dilemma

Mr C is a 46-year-old accounting clerk referred for 'assessment of symptoms related to his workplace' by his family doctor. The chief complaint is fear of exposure to toxic substances believed to be the result of racial persecution by six other employees, one of whom was previously charged with assault. Mr C was absent from work on non-medical leave with pay, due to these concerns.

The history is significant for other multiple fears of contamination. Physical examination revealed no evidence of any toxic syndrome. Mental status examination suggested possible depression. It was unclear whether his fears were based in reality, so he was referred for psychiatric assessment that subsequently confirmed a delusional disorder requiring anti-psychotic medication.

At the first visit, Mr C presented an unsolicited letter addressed directly to the treating physician from his workplace manager posing several questions regarding Mr C's medical condition and demanding the physician to respond.

The issue and resolution

The issue is one of disclosure, or entitlement to confidential information. In this case, the patient was referred by the family physician, not directly from the workplace. This was not a third party examination. Because there was no consent form signed by the patient, a letter was sent to the manager stating only that Mr C did indeed have a medical condition preventing him from working, and for which treatment was being arranged. The specific questions would not be answered.

The key learning points

In third party examinations it has been suggested that no patient-physician relationship exists, as the physician is working on behalf of the payer. Whoever pays for the examination, often an employer, owns the information and controls its release (depending on the jurisdiction), unlike an examination taking place in the medical system.

The letter from the workplace stated: "it is the policy of [this workplace] to support employees whose illness ... is affecting their ability to do their job

..." So, Mr C's manager felt entitled to know 'what was going on'. Unless the patient consents to the release of such information, however, it remains confidential. In this case, the patient did eventually sign a consent form. Only information relevant to the planning of Mr C's return to work (such as functional limitations) was divulged. His diagnosis was kept confidential.

Dr Joan Saary MD MSc
Senior Occupational Medicine Resident
St. Michael's Hospital and University of Toronto, Ontario, Canada
Medical Consultant to NASA Johnson Space Center, Texas USA

ETHICS AND LAW IN PSYCHIATRY

Dr Adrian Sutton – Manchester, England

Patrick was 11 years old when he had 'wanting to be dead feelings' again. Social Services and his school were extremely concerned about Patrick's emotional state and behaviour. Taken in conjunction with the suicidal thoughts and feelings, the information indicated a need for psychiatric assessment. To establish the level of acute risk and formulate a crisis management plan this needed to include an individual consultation. Two years earlier his father had reluctantly agreed to child psychiatric assessment and a limited intervention was possible. On this occasion Patrick's father refused to allow me to interview him.

I found myself in a dilemma. Given the risk of self-harm, should I advise Social Services to seek an Assessment Order under the Children Act to allow me to assess Patrick? However, he was fiercely loyal to his father so, if carried out with him knowing it was against his father's wishes, it could make it difficult to interpret what Patrick did or did not say. I told Patrick's father the nature of my concerns, and the possible steps open to me. He angrily told me that the judge would give the order anyway so I should just get on and see his son. I felt this would be compliance under duress, not 'informed consent', and that it could also precipitate suicidal behaviour. I was not prepared to proceed on that basis. I thought that Patrick's father's views might change given his previous partial engagement with me.

Although I was uncomfortable about judging risk without actually seeing Patrick, my prior knowledge of him and the third party information available left me thinking that he was unlikely to be at acute risk of attempting suicide and that the measures in place would protect him in the immediate situation. I decided to manage this risk while attempting to develop a co-operative approach with his father as this might have benefit in the long term. I did not immediately seek an Assessment Order and lived with the resultant anxiety and uncertainty.

Dr Adrian Sutton BSc (Hons) MB BS FRCPsych UKCP
Consultant in Child & Family Psychiatry and Psychotherapy
Central Manchester Health Care Trust
Manchester, England

ETHICS AND LAW IN GENERAL MEDICINE

Case 1 – Dr Alejandro Cragno – Buenos Aires, Argentina

Pedro is a 58-year-old man who was diagnosed with amiotrophic lateral sclerosis one year ago. He lives in Argentina, is married and has three children of school age. Pedro is a philosophy professor but has not been in work for two years. He has been unable to find work since the economic collapse of his country that has caused widespread unemployment and social exclusion.

During the past year, Pedro had been given the normal treatments, without improvement. The neurologist then informed him of a new medication that was in phase four of investigation. So far it seemed to be very effective, given the improvement that the published trials showed. The drug had been approved recently in the USA, but it had not yet been approved in Argentina. Nevertheless, the neurologist advised Pedro to ask his general practitioner to prescribe it for him.

The GP in turn, requested funding for the drug from the authorities of the Public Hospital. Despite the fact that Argentine pharmacology specialists and an eminent neurologist recognised the benefits of the drug and supported its use, the Public Hospital refused to obtain the drug. They asserted that the treatment had not been approved in Argentina, that there was little experience of the treatment; and fundamentally the lack of funds available meant that it would not be economically viable.

Pedro despaired at this decision and appealed to the highest authorities of Argentina to help him to have a chance to live, since this drug may be his only hope (though no guarantee) of survival. Ultimately the conflict was passed to the Hospital Bioethics Committee.

The dilemmas

Is it right that a society with serious economic problems prioritises funding of proven treatments over experimental ones? If a country does not have much money should it stop testing new treatments and therefore stop medical research and progress?

In situations of economic deterioration, should doctors carefully select the information they give to patients regarding treatment options? Would it have been better if the neurologist had not told Pedro about the experimental drug if Pedro was unlikely to receive it?

The outcome

Pedro finally received the drug – the laboratory provided it to him for free.

What I learnt

Nowadays in my country we have serious economic problems; the health services are in crisis. We are often faced with situations where we know that the patients have more effective treatment options but the social insurance and the public services are unable to support these financially. If there is not enough money to offer the best treatment should we, as doctors, tell the patient all the treatment options or only those that are available, even when the available treatments are not the best?

I believe the individual patient should know all the options because there are some people who may be able to pay for treatment privately, if the social insurance or public service cannot pay. From the perspective of public services, the resources must be allocated according to priorities. The problem in my country is that there are no clear rules in the health system and as a consequence there are permanent conflicts between the managers and people.

Dr Alejandro Cragno MD
Consultant Physician
Bahía Blanca Medical Association Hospital
Buenos Aires, Argentina

Case 2 – Dr Anthony Toft – Edinburgh, Scotland

The dilemma

A 43-year-old woman presented with a three-month history of secondary amenorrhoea, heat intolerance and palpitations. Among various investigations raised serum total thyroxine and low thyrotrophin concentrations were found, consistent with a diagnosis of hyperthyroidism.

She was referred for treatment with iodine-131 when clinical examination detected a small but diffusely enlarged thyroid and isotope studies were in keeping with a diagnosis of Graves' disease. She received 400 MBq iodine-131 and three weeks later was found to be 16 weeks pregnant. The fetal thyroid could have been capable of concentrating radioiodine at the time of therapy and there was, therefore, a risk of fetal hypothyroidism and neuropsychological disadvantage.

Difficult issues

Routine advice would be to recommend termination of pregnancy, particularly as there had been five previously successful pregnancies and this latest was unplanned. The patient refused the option of abortion. It later transpired that a pregnancy test had been requested as part of the initial investigations by the GP but had wrongly been reported to the patient as negative.

What was done

Monitoring was carried out by measuring thyroxine and thyrotrophin in fetal blood obtained by cordocentesis with a view to treatment with intra-amniotic thyroxine in the event of evidence of thyroid failure. Fortunately, fetal thyroid function was normal throughout pregnancy and at routine neonatal screening at five days. Subsequent development has been normal.

What has been learnt

The issue is whether pregnancy testing should be routine in women of child-bearing age before treatment with iodine-131. It has been thought sufficient to provide written and verbal warnings to patients of the contra-indication to iodine-131 treatment if pregnant or planning pregnancy within four months. Whether this case, the first example of the inadvertent use of iodine-131 during pregnancy in our patient clinic in more than 5,000 patients over the age of 35 years should alter our policy, is debatable. In the index patient, of course, pregnancy testing did not prevent the inappropriate use of radioactive iodine.

Dr Anthony Toft CBE FRCP
Consultant Endocrinologist
Royal Infirmary
Edinburgh, Scotland

Case 3 – Dr Shrilla Banerjee & Dr Peter Mills – London, England

The dilemma

Mrs GW is an 81-year-old widowed lady who lives independently and is accompanied by her married daughter. While out shopping, she collapses and is brought to hospital via ambulance. She gives a history of breathlessness, followed by light-headedness, preceding the collapse. On examination, she has a blood pressure of 130/90, and a loud ejection systolic murmur with a thrill in the aortic area. The murmur radiates to the carotid arteries.

Blood tests reveal renal dysfunction with a creatinine of 185 μmol/L, and a microcytic anaemia (Haemoglobin10.6 g/dL with a mean cell volume of 67 fL). All other blood tests are normal. Faecal occult bloods are positive and she gives a history of alteration of her bowel habit in the last three months. Echocardiography confirms aortic stenosis with a calculated Doppler gradient of 100 mm Hg. She has severe aortic stenosis, mild renal failure and a micro-cytic anaemia possibly related to a large bowel carcinoma.

Her daughter is concerned that her mother may lose her independence and is anxious that she should undergo cardiac surgery. What management should be considered?

Difficult issues

This lady would benefit from Aortic Valve Replacement (AVR). However, her co-morbidities will put her at increased risk from the operation. The suggested mortality from AVR in the over 80's is 8.5%. (Kohl P, Kerzmann A, Lahaye L, Gerard P, Limet R. Cardiac surgery in octogenarians: peri-operative outcome and long-term results. *European Heart Journal* 2001 Jul; 22(14): 1235–43.) However, her renal dysfunction will increase her operative risk and may worsen during the post-operative period and require dialysis, possibly permanently. In addition, she will require further investigation of anaemia and change of bowel habit before cardiac surgery. She will also need to undergo coronary angiography to determine whether or not she has coexisting coronary disease that will further increase her operative risk.

The management

This patient went on to have the AVR after discussion with the consultant surgeon and cardiologist. She had a stormy post-operative course and required dialysis for two weeks, but was eventually discharged home well. Her anaemia was found to be related to an adenoma, which was removed at colonoscopy (covered with antibiotics). She will require surveillance colonoscopy at six-monthly intervals. She is now living independently once more.

The important learning point

The important point here is that as the patient was independent and mentally competent before her admission, the management options must be discussed with her. In the first instance she needs to be aware of the risks and benefits of any surgical intervention for aortic stenosis. She should be allowed to judge whether she feels the procedure is appropriate and wishes to be considered for surgery. While it is helpful to include her daughter in these discussions, informed consent is essential in this situation and she should meet the surgeon, so both may evaluate each other. The risks of not having the procedure done should also be defined, as there is a high risk of sudden death in this population, if left untreated.

The final decision about surgery can only be made once the results of all relevant investigations are available. Do not assume that because her daughter wants the patient to have an operation that the patient herself will agree to major surgery.

Dr Shrilla Bannerjee MB ChB MD MRCP
Specialist Registrar in Cardiology

Dr Peter Mills BM BSc FRCP
Consultant Cardiologist

The Royal London Hospital
London, England

ETHICS AND LAW IN SPORTS MEDICINE

Dr Vassilis Lykomitros – Athens, Greece

The dilemma

A 21-year-old athlete was preparing to compete in the Olympic Games as a member of his national rowing team. During the mandatory pre-participation testing, a dysfunction in the cardiac conduction pathways was revealed. The athlete underwent further electrophysiological studies under sedation that showed an arrhythmic electric destabilisation.

The professor who conducted the test said that there was a slight chance that he could have a cardiac arrest during exertion or stress, stating as an example, that he would never allow this athlete to pilot an aeroplane.

Despite the risk of suffering a fatal arrhythmia during intensive exercise, the athlete insisted that he should still be allowed to race in the Olympic Games. He argued that he had never experienced any symptoms before, despite much training and competition in previous years. He was otherwise completely healthy and his family history was also negative.

During multidisciplinary meetings with other colleagues the idea of introducing a pacemaker in the athlete's body was discussed. This could, in theory, prevent episodes of arrhythmias from occurring. However there was nothing in the international literature to show that this had been tried before, nor of any other solution which would allow him to continue sporting activities.

What issues made it difficult?

- A laboratory test revealed a potential problem but clinically the athlete was asymptomatic, even during extreme exertion training for international competition.
- The athlete insisted that he be allowed to race – he was ready to put his life in danger because the Olympic Games were his dream and life ambition.
- All the Government authorities (Secretary of Sports, Rowing Federation, club, sports centre) refused to take responsibility for the ultimate decision, leaving it completely up to me as team doctor.
- The Federation and Government refused the idea of introducing a pacemaker because it was too politically risky. They were worried about the negative press and public reaction which could result if it was discovered that athletes were encouraged to risk their lives representing the nation.

What I did

I decided to withdraw the athlete from the national team and the sport, but I could not persuade him to stop his private sporting life and continue a sedative life in the future. This was very difficult for me because I know from personal experience that as a professional athlete you live for the excitement of competing, and the pride of representing your country. At international level, the sport takes over your life to the exclusion of nearly everything else, and you feel that if you cannot compete, your life is over.

What did I learn from it?

I learned that as an individual person you can do whatever you want with your life but as a member of a team you have to protect both yourself and the other team members.

Young people may be ready to give their lives for ideals but experienced people need to guide them by explaining facts. When you have the responsibility, sometimes you need to make hard decisions to protect human lives as the Hippocratic Oath states.

I regret that I hesitated about introducing a pacemaker in this athlete, which could have allowed him to compete and continue his career. However, this seemed a difficult road to take at the time because there was no international precedent. Four years later there are now two papers from other countries describing the introduction of pacemakers in fine athletes in similar cases.

Dr Vassilis Lykomitros MD
Orthopaedic Spinal Surgeon
Former Olympic athlete – Greek Rowing Team
Manager of Rowing, 2004 Olympic Games
Athens, Greece

ETHICS AND LAW IN PAEDIATRICS

Case 1 – Dr Jamiu Busari – Curaçao, Netherlands Antilles

The dilemma:

A 38-year-old primigravida delivered a female premature neonate. Shortly after birth, the baby was transfused with erythrocytes due to an acute anaemia. The mother's obstetrical history revealed three previous pregnancies, two of which resulted in spontaneous abortions and a third in a stillbirth. Due to her obstetrical history and age, she had requested to see an obstetrician for antenatal screening for fetal congenital abnormalities. The obstetrician reassured her that despite her obstetrical history, the pregnancy was not at risk. No antenatal screening tests had been performed.

In addition to the child's anaemia, on physical examination, dysmorphological physical features were found. An ultrasonography and CT scan of the brain revealed extensive (grade IV) intra-cerebral bleeding. An echocardiogram of the heart revealed an open foramen ovale as the only abnormal finding.

The parents were so happy with this baby after all the previous (unfruitful) attempts at bearing a child. Sadly, they were informed of the baby's clinical condition and the poor prognosis. The decision was made to discontinue active medical intervention. Supportive care and comfort was provided until the baby's demise two weeks later.

What made the issues difficult?

- Convincing the parents about our decision (based on medical grounds) to discontinue treatment. A conflict arose between the moral views on life and death, and my professional responsibility to act in the patient's best interest, which was to discontinue intensive treatment in this case. As a physician, the decision to abstain from active medical intervention was based on the poor prognosis of the child's situation and the consensus from the collaboration with colleagues in allied disciplines. A second problem was informing the parents that intensive treatment was being discontinued knowing how dear this pregnancy and child was to them.
- Convincing the parents (who were devout Christians) of the poor prognosis of their daughter's condition. Although the parents appeared to understand the severity of the situation from the medical point of view, they still held a strong belief that a miracle would happen and heal

their daughter. It was difficult convincing them of the child's poor prognosis.

- Following the decision to abstain from further intensive medical care, the child received a second blood transfusion. This was because I believed that it was inhumane not to give blood knowing the child was anaemic. In addition, a second CT scan of the brain was performed in order to re-assess the degree of the intra-cerebral haemorrhage.

What I did

- Ensured careful and detailed documentation of each meeting with the parents by both the nursing and medical staff.
- Acknowledged the parent's religious views and an attempt was made to have the parents meet the hospital's pastor for support.
- Upon my request, the clinical plan was re-examined and the medical orders clearly stated again. This was to avoid (more) confusion or send conflicting messages to the parents that could falsely raise their hopes.

What I learnt from it

- A great degree of understanding, compassion and empathy should be exhibited in such circumstances.
- The views of the patient (in this case the parents) should be acknowledged, even when they are in conflict with medical findings. The intervention of allied services (e.g. pastoral) can be beneficial in such circumstances.
- There should be strict adherence to the medical plan after extensive multidisciplinary collaboration and consensus.

Dr Jamiu Busari MD MHPE
Specialist registrar in Paediatrics
St. Elisabeth Hospital
Curaçao, Netherlands Antilles

Case 2 – Professor Marcellina Mian – Toronto, Canada

Four-year-old Jennifer was wheelchair-bound because of severe weakness due to thalassemia with a haemoglobin of 4mg/L. Her parents, Jehovah's Witnesses, had refused periodic transfusions and would not consent to splenectomy for Jennifer as the surgeon and anaesthesiologist would not do the surgery without a pre-operative transfusion to raise her haemoglobin into a safer range. The parents would allow the surgery if the physicians agreed to transfusing the child only if she decompensated intraoperatively. Through their network, the parents obtained the agreement from physicians at a smaller institution to do the surgery without transfusing Jennifer beforehand. Our dilemma was whether to allow her transfer or to notify the child protection authorities of the fact that Jennifer's life and well-being were being placed at increased risk.

The issues

- Relative weight of spiritual and physical dictates in deciding on a child's best interest.
- Defining limits of parental right to choose the level of risk to which a child's life can be exposed.

Ontario child welfare law requires reporting of situations where a child's safety and well-being may be at risk. Accordingly, we reported the parents' plan to the authorities, giving the opinion that it would increase the child's risk of complications, including death, unacceptably (estimatedly from about 2 to 10%). After hearing from all concerned, the authorities allowed the surgery without elective transfusion. Jennifer did well.

The lesson learned was an appreciation of the subjectivity of risk-taking thresholds. Further, this case demonstrated the difficulty of promoting safe practice. The favourable resolution in this case did not affect the basic dilemma and is not likely to affect future practice. An unfavourable outcome, however, would have affected both health and social practice for the future in terms of placing greater emphasis on the need to safeguard the child's physical well-being.

Professor Marcellina Mian MDCM FRCPC
Associate Professor of Paediatrics
University of Toronto
Ontario, Canada

Case 3 – Dr Hamish Wallace & Dr Elizabeth Morris – Edinburgh, Scotland

The dilemma

A nine-year-old girl called Emma had presented with acute lymphoblastic leukaemia two years ago. Emma had acute lymphoblastic leukaemia that initially responded poorly to treatment. In addition, she had an abnormal chromosome pattern within the leukaemia cells, and for these two reasons, deemed to be high risk. She was switched to a more intensive induction therapy and eventually did achieve remission, but unfortunately, after 14 months of treatment she developed back pain and a limp.

As these were similar symptoms to those at presentation, her bone marrow was examined and this confirmed relapsed acute lymphoblastic leukaemia. There was no evidence of central nervous system disease at presentation or at relapse. During her 14 months of treatment there had been a number of admissions to hospital with side effects of treatment, which the family had found extremely difficult and distressing.

The outlook for a young girl, who relapses 14 months into treatment, is extremely poor. Conventional practice in this situation is to give further intensive chemotherapy with a view to achieving a second stable bone marrow remission. This would be followed with total body irradiation and an allogeneic bone marrow transplant from either her sister or a matched unrelated donor.

The chances of achieving remission in this situation are at least 50%, but the chances of long term cure of the disease after relapse while on chemotherapy are poor, and certainly less than 10%.

Further chemotherapy treatment would put her at high risk of developing infections, sore mouth and diarrhoea. Even if she should go into remission with intensive chemotherapy, the side effects of total body irradiation would include a premature menopause with a life-long requirement for hormone replacement therapy and little or no chance, even with donated eggs, of carrying a pregnancy to term.

After discussion with the medical team, Emma's parents decided that their daughter had suffered enough and she should not receive further chemotherapy. They were concerned about the side effects of treatment and did not want to put Emma through a bone marrow transplant with all the short, medium and long-term side effects that this was likely to entail. Emma's parents consulted widely, including their Jesuit priest who agreed that they were making the correct decision, but the physician responsible for her care was unhappy with this.

The legal context

In the UK, a young person of 16 years or over is presumed to be capable of giving legally valid consent to treatment. A child or young person under 16 is presumed not to be capable of giving legally valid consent, but may be able to demonstrate that they are capable of doing so if they can show that they understand the implications of what they are consenting to. In the case of the child or young person under the age of 16 who is not deemed competent, the parents can give proxy consent to medical procedures which are considered to be 'in the best interests' of their child. It is the 'best interests' test for medical interventions, treatments and procedures that governs the right of parents to give proxy consent on behalf of their children for treatment.

Summary of ethical issues

In this case, the clinical team was faced with a 10-year-old girl who had leukaemia which had relapsed after 14 months of treatment, and whose parents had refused consent to further chemotherapy.

This is an unusual dilemma, which has serious ethical ramifications. Most parents in this situation would be happy to give consent to further treatment of their child, bearing in mind the chance of achieving a stable remission and the small (less than 10%) chance of achieving a cure. Is it in her 'best interests' for Emma to have further treatment with all the side effects that may be entailed, or to move straight into a palliative care phase where the likelihood of death due to recurrent disease is only a few weeks away?

Are Emma's parents in a sufficiently strong ethical position to deny their daughter further treatment, on the basis of the 'best interests' test? Is Emma, who is now aged 10 years, able to go against the wishes of her parents and give informed consent for further treatment? Are the medical and nursing teams able to give Emma further treatment against her parents' wishes, believing it is in the best interests of Emma to receive further medical intervention?

What actually happened?

It became clear that Emma herself had not been given the opportunity to decide whether she wanted further treatment or not. It is, of course, a natural reaction for parents to be protective of their children and very often they are keen for words like 'cancer' and 'leukaemia' to be avoided at all costs in discussions with the patients themselves.

Further discussion with Emma's parents allowed them to let Emma herself enter the debate. While it was clear that Emma had experienced significant side effects during her first 14 months of treatment, she was not concerned about receiving further chemotherapy and even progressing towards a bone marrow transplant. Once she had become an active participant in the treatment decisions, it became quite clear that she wanted to have further treatment.

The opening up of the ethical debate to include the patient herself, although she was only 10 years old (and certainly well below the legal age of consent), enabled her parents, the medical and nursing staff to come to a firm decision about further treatment that everybody felt happy with.

Emma received further intensive chemotherapy. She was hospitalised and required intravenous antibiotics, and during this period of time she was not particularly unwell. Five weeks into this second line treatment, her bone marrow was examined and unfortunately did not show remission. In view of the fact that it was now extremely unlikely that a further block of treatment would achieve a stable remission and allow progression to bone marrow transplant, treatment was discontinued and she was discharged home for palliative care. Sadly she died two weeks after going home.

Learning points

Young people under the age of 16 are not legally considered to be able to give valid consent to medical treatment, but are often able to understand the issues involved and give informed consent for further treatment if allowed to participate in the treatment discussions. Young patients should never be excluded from treatment discussions and they should be given the opportunity to become involved. It is essential that discussions take place in a language that they themselves can understand. In our experience, young people will often have strong views about their treatment, show great understanding of the issues, and give a lead to both their parents and the medical and nursing staff responsible for their care.

Dr Hamish Wallace MD FRCPCH FRCP(Edin)
Consultant Paediatric Oncologist
Royal Hospital for Sick Children
Edinburgh, Scotland

Dr Elizabeth Morris MB ChB MRCGP
General Practitioner
Edinburgh, Scotland

ETHICS AND LAW IN INTENSIVE CARE

Case 1 – Dr Bob Taylor – Belfast, Northern Ireland

A nine-year-old boy presented with a severe brain injury as the result of an accident. Five days following his admission to a paediatric intensive care unit, appropriate tests confirmed brainstem death. Despite being given explanatory information by the medical and nursing staff the child's father refused to permit the doctors to switch off the ventilator. Other options for management including withdrawing or withholding treatment were discussed by the doctors and the parents. These, however, were also refused.

Despite many hours of explanation, persuasion and argument it proved impossible to obtain the approval of the father to discontinue ventilation. It was unclear whether the father had any legal rights in this matter. Again, several options were discussed, including stopping ventilation in any case. Despite the recognition that stopping ventilation at this stage, after brainstem death had been confirmed, would not result in criminal charges against the doctors, it appeared that the best option would be to continue ventilation until the situation could be resolved.

Good relations were maintained with both parents and it was accepted that they both had similar, if not equal, rights to consent for the minor but that the refusal of one parent outweighed the consent of the other. Therefore, with the agreement of both parents, social services were requested to seek wardship of the minor. This would clarify parental responsibility, ensure privacy and permit a court decision regarding withdrawal of artificial ventilation.

An emergency High Court sitting was arranged four days after formal brainstem tests had confirmed death. The trust applied to the court for wardship of the minor to be awarded to the local authority and to confirm that brainstem death equated to death. On the second court day the father contacted the doctors and requested that ventilation be terminated. The hospital trust therefore requested the court's permission to withdraw its application. This was granted which effectively left the decision to discontinue ventilation back in the hands of the doctors and parents. The ventilator was switched off that same day, five days after the child had been declared brainstem dead.

Dr RH Taylor MA MB FFARCSI
Consultant Paediatric Anaesthetist and Director of Paediatric Intensive Care,
Royal Belfast Hospital for Sick Children
Belfast, Northern Ireland

Case 2 – Dr Stephen Child – Auckland, New Zealand

In late January this year, an 81–year-old lady was admitted to the medical ward with a 24–hour history of vomiting. She had no significant co-morbidity apart from mild osteoarthritis. She was subsequently found to be hypotensive and mildly hypoxic (oxygen saturation of 90%). Blood tests showed: Platelets $72x10^9$/L, mildly elevated Liver Function Tests (LFTs) and a Creatinine of 180μol/L with oliguria of 220 ml/24 hours. Our working diagnosis was one of sepsis (subsequently proven correct with positive (Klebsiella Pneumonia) blood cultures) with multi-organ failure and Acute Renal Failure secondary to Acute Tubular Necrosis (ATN).

We gave her fluids, inotropes, oxygen and antibiotics and asked our intensive care unit (ICU) to see her for haemodynamic monitoring and potential dialysis or respiratory support if it became necessary. Our intensive care unit replied that she was 'too sick' and that her poor prognosis precluded her admission to ICU.

We were then faced with the difficult dilemma of explaining to the family that their mother was too sick for us to 'try' to save her! I was furious. I knew that the literature for sepsis with 3 organ failure and ATN states that she was facing a risk of 70% mortality but I did not accept that the ICU could protect their resources in this way and not accept a patient on these grounds.

To make the matter more interesting, the actual issue arose because we had also consulted the surgeons about her abdominal pain. They had responded that we should do a CT of her abdomen – and if it showed a drainable collection then they would see her, but if not then she was not surgical. ICU initially said that they would take her if she went to theatre but not if she didn't!

So what did we do?

First of all, I had an open discussion with my registrar, reviewing the medical facts and treatment options. I then expressed my opinion and we discussed our approach together to the family. We tried to get ICU to talk to the son directly but they refused so my registrar eventually spoke to the son and outlined the likely futility of our actions anyway.

I spoke to the ICU consultant and flagged the case for our Quality Review. As I remained unsatisfied, I then presented this case to our hospital grand rounds and invited ICU to comment. The lecture theatre was packed with over 150 doctors and we had an excellent discussion on the topic. Essentially ICU continued to defend its decision based primarily on resources and all agreed to improve the communications between ICU and other hospital staff.

The woman did go into complete renal failure and was provided with palliative care from Day 5. She died peacefully with her family at her side on Day 11 of her hospital stay.

Dr Stephen Child MD FRCP(C) FRACP
Consultant Physician and Director of Clinical Training
Auckland Hospital
Auckland, New Zealand

Case 3 – Professor Graham Ramsay – Maastricht, The Netherlands
         Dr Francesca Rubulotta and Associate Professor Mitchell Levy
         – Providence (RI), USA

Case description

A 79-year-old white woman initially presented with osteomyelitis in the lumbar spine (L1–L2) and received long-term intravenous antibiotics, and oral opioids for lumbar back pain relief. The patient lived alone and at home she developed shortness of breath, palpitations, left arm swelling and pain. After three days she presented in the emergency room where she was found to be hypoxic and with atrial fibrillation. Past medical history included hypertension, diabetes mellitus, atrial fibrillation, atherosclerotic heart disease, and peripheral vascular disease.

The patient was transferred to the Respiratory Intensive Care Unit, where she was sedated, intubated, ventilated, and a central line was placed via her left jugular vein. Her skin was cool and dry, and she had no fever or oedema. Her chest radiograph showed left lower lobe infiltrates and the ECG normal sinus rhythm with a rate of 140 beats/min. She received medication for heart rate control, and the left central venous line was removed and cultured. The patient was successfully weaned off the ventilator but the ICU course was complicated by left subclavian-brachio-cephalic vein thrombosis and nosocomial pneumonia. Over the 12 hours after the extubation she developed hypotension, hyponatremia and respiratory alkalosis. She was transferred to the Medical Intensive Care Unit (MICU) with the diagnosis of acute hypoxic respiratory failure and pneumonia in a patient with a high risk for pulmonary embolism. Her chest x-ray showed pulmonary infiltrates highly suggestive, while the CT pulmonary angiography was negative, for pulmonary embolism. Seven days later the patient was successfully weaned and transferred, alert and orientated, to a general ward.

She was probably discharged too early from the ICU and after 24 hours she was found to be lethargic with an arterial pH of 7.19. She was re-intubated for hypercarbic respiratory failure and re-admitted to the ICU where her systolic blood pressure dropped to 80mmHg and white blood count rose to 31×10^9/L. She developed a left knee effusion, right upper extremity cellulitis, right internal jugular line infection, and septic shock. Noradrenaline was started and continued for five days, to maintain normal blood pressure. The patient had fever and a new chest x-ray showed extensive bilateral infiltrates, partial right mid and lower lobe collapse, atelectasis with a possible malignant mass. The CT scan revealed changes in the posterior wall of a right intermediate bronchus. A bronchoscopy with broncho-alveolar lavage (BAL) and brushings of the right mid lobe was performed revealing neither a clear source of pneumonia nor neoplastic cells. The vasopressor was gradually stopped, while bilirubin, urea, nitrate and creatinine continuously worsened from baseline levels. The arterial blood gas indicated significant metabolic acidosis and urine output decreased to less than 5 ml/h.

Over the next three days she worsened with pneumonia, sepsis, renal failure, increased pleural effusions, and pancytopenia. There was neither a living will, nor advance directives on the chart. The patient was clearly incompetent to voice her wishes. Her relatives were contacted and the situation was explained to them for the first time in detail. The two daughters participated together as patient's surrogate in the difficult process of decision making. They realised the poor prognosis, and as they already had had a similar experience with their father they knew, from earlier discussions at home, that their mother would not have prolonged this situation. They asked to have her as comfortable as possible and the code status changed from Full Measures to Comfort Measures Only (CMO). The patient was extubated and her breathing appeared laboured. To keep the patient comfortable intravenous morphine was started at 5 mg/h and titrated up to 7mg/h. Her breathing became irregular and stopped. Her family remained quietly with her for a period after death was declared.

Learning questions

Is palliative care fully adopted in intensive care units?

Despite advances in critical care medicine and in outcome research, death continues to be common in the ICU and less predictable than in the past decade.[1] In the case of the present patient the combination of multiple medical problems and rapidly changing clinical status makes predicting outcome a very difficult task. Many ICU patients die while still receiving aggressive interventions to extend life. A major challenge in hospital care is identifying better ways to cure illness while avoiding needless physical and emotional harm to terminal patients. The idea that palliative care should be detached from Intensive Care is no longer tenable. The main reason is that over the last century death has moved out of homes, and withholding or withdrawal of life-support is becoming a common way of dying. An enormous amount of healthcare resources are delivered to dying patients,[2] and the considerable number of intensive interventions used before death is a troubling finding that critics argued might be appropriate and consistent with patients' wishes. Currently about 60% of Americans die in an acute care unit[3] but 90% of them would want to die at home.[4] Nearly half of all patients who die in the hospital are transferred to an ICU three days before death and the incidence of distress and discomfort seems to increase proportionally to aggressive care administration.

Should we gradually shift from aggressive therapies to palliative care or accept a sudden change from full code to CMO?

The ineffectiveness in determining the timing for the shift from primarily curative care to primarily palliative care is the main reason why the current patient received numerous invasive and expensive procedures just before death. The BAL performed the evening before withdrawing care would be useful looking for lung carcinoma to aid the decision. This invasive low risk procedure would not improve or change the patient's treatment. There is an open question whether this or even other invasive exams are necessary to make a correct decision in end of life scenarios. Numerous obstacles may limit optimal palliative care in ICUs, such as the lack of sensitive or specific tools to assess patients' outcome or inadequate training of professional caregivers. In the case of the present patient we can state that uncertainty about the prognosis was the major barrier to optimal palliative care planning. The disease worsened extremely rapidly and left little time to gradually shift from cure to care measures. This situation is very common when treating critical diseases suggesting the need to join palliative care with critical care medicine. In modern ICUs one patient should opportunely or alternatively receive aggressive palliation or aggressive resuscitation.

Data suggest unacceptable levels of suffering during ICU treatments, and several authors argue that much more can be done to relieve pain and anxiety, to respect personal dignity, and to provide opportunities for people finding meaning in life's conclusion.[5,6,7] Physicians should realise that there are many routine procedures that may cause unnecessary discomfort to hospitalised dying patients such as daily laboratory tests, regular radiographic examinations, and frequent determination of vital signs. Distressing symptoms are underestimated by caregivers, even if they are associated with unfavourable outcomes such as a higher mortality.[8] There is no evidence that prevention of patient suffering would compromise aggressive efforts to prolong life, while the lack of pain and anxiety relief may limit the possibility of weaning and rehabilitating a patient. In one study[6] authors showed that unrelieved distressing symptoms are present even in an ICU where their management is a major focus of attention.

What would be the right time for the first meeting?

The lack of an appropriate relationship between the patient, her surrogates and the caregiver has characterised the management of the present case. Communication with families in the intensive care setting is difficult. Clinicians, counsellors, ethicists, researchers, and lawyers are studying in the attempt to guide how to hold meetings regarding life-sustaining issues.

Effective communication is a skill composed by several humanistic qualities such as compassion, empathy, and sensitivity. Both physicians and nurses working in an ICU need some general principles of patient-clinician relationship and trust. As stated Prof. Levy (co-writer): "Unfortunately for our patients, the irony is that just because we see death all the time we are not necessarily comfortable with it."

Physicians cannot assume that patients or families will wish to plan death explicitly or will want to be actively involved in end-of-life care assessments. The result of one study showed that when the attending physician adequately communicates with families more preferences are documented in the medical record and resource utilization is decreased.[15] In the case of the present patient ICU staff should have informed the family of the severity of the prognostic panel before the last admission. The relationship with patients and families is a new duty ICU physicians have to routinely accomplish to correctly adapt his or her therapy to the scenario. A national survey of 80% of US academic centres found that students, residents, and academic leaders evaluate themselves as inadequately prepared to provide compassionate end-of-life care.[16]

The implementation of a programme for training residents on ethical issues has impact on patients' treatment and length of ICU stay for both survivors and non-survivors.[14] A significant proportion of people are not familiar with instruments such as living wills or durable powers of attorney. Fortunately the surrogates in this case had a previous experience and had discussed end-of-life preferences with their loved one before this hospitalisation. A meeting with the patient after her first extubation or before her discharge from the ICU, or even with her family, would have improved resources allocation, and above all the patient's compassionate care.

What would be the right number of meetings and the right amount of information?

One very important principle of compassionate care is that preferences and goals may change as an illness progresses. ICU patients often lose the capacity of decision-making during their hospitalisation, and surrogates do not always accurately reflect the right preferences. For this reason ideally patient-physician meetings should not be a single event. The severity of critical illnesses does not leave enough time to meet patients or relatives more than once. Physicians need to be confident about what the patient's prognosis would be, before asking what 'he or she would like to receive as treatment'. This is a reasonable concept knowing that the same patient may receive full aggressive intensive care from one healthcare provider and only comfort measure from another.[9]

May a previous family meeting shorten hospitalisation (the proxy had a similar experience in the past and knew the patient's wishes)?

Before holding a family meeting the physician should focus on what he or she would suggest as code status (resuscitation status). Dramatic differences in judgments are recorded in a large survey in Canada asking physicians and nurses about the appropriate level of care for patients presented in different scenarios.[10] In the current literature the incidence of patients dying with full aggressive measures in place may range from 4% to 79%, while the incidence of withdrawing life-support ranges from 0 to 79% with a high variability existing between world ICUs. We may assume that the lack of an earlier meeting in the case presented would not necessarily have reduced the length of her ICU or hospital stay.

Should physicians admit this patient again in the MICU?

The possibility to re-admit a patient is related to the specific ICU setting. Bed availability, for example, is the major factor in the use of intensive care in Spain, Portugal and United Kingdom.

Was the last intubation strictly necessary?

The SUPPORT trial showed that a substantial majority of patients have not discussed preferences for life-sustaining treatment even after 14 days of hospitalisation.[11] A large survey among several American Thoracic Critical Care Units[12] reported that 34% of physicians continued life-sustaining treatments despite patients' or surrogates' wishes, and 25% of those who withheld or withdrew care did so without consent, and 14% without even the knowledge of patients or their surrogates. The percentage of patients with some kind of advance directive is about 10% in the United States, and those who had such directives are more likely to have documented orders or code status in their medical records. According to some authors nearly 70% of patients have some restrictions on care before death.[13]

Conclusion

The dying process involves the healthcare system more and more and as a consequence physicians need to acquire end-of-life skills. To constantly involve patients and surrogates in the decision making process is a duty of modern ICU staff. Knowledge of the ongoing fusion between intensive care and palliative care is leading to new resource allocation and changing therapeutic goals.

Professor Graham Ramsay MD PhD FRCS
Chairman of Intensive Care
University Hospital (Academisch Ziekenhuis)
Maastricht, The Netherlands

Dr Francesca Rubulotta MD
Research Fellow
Brown University
Providence
Rhode Island, USA

Associate Professor Mitchell Levy MD
Chairman of Intensive Care
Brown University
Providence
Rhode Island, USA

References

1. Nelson JE, Danis M. End-life care in the intensive care unit: Where are we now? *Crit Care Med* 2001; 29:N2–N9
2. Cher DJ, Lenert LA. Method of Medicare reimbursement and the rate of potentially ineffective care of critically ill patients. *JAMA* 2001; 278:1001–1007
3. Field M, Cassel C. Approaching Death improving Care at the End of Life. (Washington DC: National Academy Press, 1997)
4. Knowledge and Attitudes related to Hospice Care National Hospice Organization Survey. The Gallup Organization. (Princeton, NJ: Gallup Organization, 1996)
5. Somogyi-Zalud E, Zhong Z, Lynn J. Dying with acute respiratory failure or multiple organ system failure with sepsis. *J Am Geriatr Soc* 2000; 48:S140–S145
6. Nelson JE, Meier DE, Oei EJ. The symptom experience of critically ill cancer patients receiving intensive care. *Crit Care Med* 2001
7. Nelson JE, Meier DE. Palliative care in the intensive care unit. *J Int Care Med* 1999; 14:130–139, 189–199
8. Chang VT, Thaler HT, Plyak HT. Quality of life and survival. *Cancer* 1998; 83:173–179

9. Cook DJ, Guyatt HG, Jaeschke R. Determinants in Canadian health care workers of the decision to withdraw life support from the critically ill. *JAMA* 1995; 273:703–709

10. Kolef MH. Private attending physician status and the withdrawal of life-sustaining interventions in a medical intensive care unit population. *Crit Care Med* 1996; 24:968–975

11. SUPPORT: A controlled trial to improve care for seriously ill hospital-ized patients. *JAMA* 1995; 274:1591–1598

12. Asch DA, Hansen-Flaschen J, Lanken P. Decisions to limit or continue life-sustaining treatment by critical care physicians in the United States: Conflicts between physicians' practice and patients' wishes. *Am J Respir Crit Care Med* 1995; 151:288–292

13. Prendergast TJ, Claessen MT, Luce JM. A national survey of end-life care for critically ill patients. *Am J Resp Crit Care Med* 1998; 158:1163–7

14. Holloran SD, Strakey GW, Burke PA. An educational intervention in the surgical intensive care unit to improve clinical decisions. *Surgery* 1995; 118:294–299

15. Dowdy MD, Robertson C, Bander JA. A study of proactive ethics consultation for critically and terminally ill patients with extended length of stay. *Crit Care Med* 1998; 26:252–259.

16. Block SD, Sullivan AM. Attitudes about end of life care: a national cross sectional study. *J Palliat Med* 1998; 1:347–355

ETHICS AND LAW IN SURGERY

Dr Nermin Halkic & Professor Michel Gillet – Lausanne, Switzerland

A 36-year-old mother of two young children was admitted to the medical intensive care unit with a fulminant hepatitis of unknown origin. Consistent with this diagnosis, she had hepatic encephalopathy, a coagulopathy, and factor V of 42 % (normal range 70–140%).

Immunological tests revealed that she had chronic hepatitis B (HBV) in the reactivation phase. The reactivation was on a background of HIV with a viral-load of 350,000 molecules/ml (>100,000/ml is very high), and a CD4 count of $180x10^6$/L (normal range $700–1500x10^6$/L). The general condition of the patient quickly worsened and the surgeon was faced with the decision of whether to carry out a liver transplant or not, knowing that this would be her only chance of survival.

The surgical team decided to go ahead and immediately carried out an orthotopic liver transplant. No major complications resulted and she has remained well since the operation, seven months ago.

This case re-ignited an already open discussion in all transplant centres, concerning organ transplantation in patients with HIV. It is not logical to transplant an organ into a patient in the terminal phase of HIV, for the same reasons as it is inappropriate to transplant an organ into a patient with chronic multi-metastatic hepatic carcinoma[1] because despite the procedure the prognosis is poor (life expectancy is only a few months). However, since the introduction of anti-retroviral triple therapy, the survival of HIV patients has greatly improved. It is also now possible to control the incidence of opportunistic infections (the principle cause of death) in patients with chronic HIV.[1,2] Until now, only 40 cases of liver transplantation in HIV patients have been described in the literature. The mean survival time of these patients is 36 months, with a range of 3 months to 12 years.[3]

In view of the speed of development in anti-retroviral therapy, we believe there is a place for transplantation in patients with HIV, despite the current paucity of organs in Europe. We believe that transplant teams should learn from our American colleagues; and make a complete revision of their restrictive attitude and discrimination policy against HIV patients who, in the coming years, could benefit from curative treatments.[1,4] HIV positive patients who are otherwise well should be considered as normal patients with regard to all medical interventions, including organ transplantation.[5]

Dr Nermin Halkic MD
Chef de Clinique

Professor Michel Gillet MD
Chef du Service

Department of Surgery
University Hospital (Centre Hospitalier Universitaire Vaudois)
Lausanne, Switzerland

References

1. Halpern SD, Ubel PA, Caplan AL. Solid-organ transplantation in HIV-infected patients. *New England Journal of Medicine* 2002; 25;347:284–7
2. Roland M, Carlson L, Stock P. Solid organ transplantation in HIV-infected individuals. *AIDS Clin Care* 2002; 14:59–63
3. Stock P, Roland M, Carlson L, et al. Solid organ transplantation in HIV-positive patients. *Transplant Proc* 2001 Nov-Dec; 33(7–8):3646–8
4. Prachalias AA, Pozniak A. Taylor et al. Liver transplantation in adults coinfected with HIV. *Transplantation* 2001 Nov 27; 72(10):1684–8
5. Gow PJ, Pillay D, Mutimer D. Solid organ transplantation in patients with HIV infection. *Transplantation* 2001 Jul 27; 72(2):177–81

USING PATIENTS' COMPLAINTS TO IMPROVE CARE

Associate Professor Merrilyn Walton – Sydney, Australia

The benefits of patients' complaints are only now being appreciated. Along with incident monitoring systems complaints inform us about problems in the way healthcare is delivered. Individually and collectively they indicate areas for improvement.

The vast majority of complaints to complaint authorities and hospitals relate to diagnosis and treatment. Mistakes made in the care and treatment of patients are not usually the 'fault' of any one person but a result of the system of care in which patients are treated. While a patient may complain about a particular medical student or doctor, an analysis of the complaint will usually discover many factors involved in the patient's care and treatment. Some doctors think a defensive attitude is the best approach to complaints but studies (see references at the end of this chapter) show that patients are more likely to complain and sue doctors when there is no apology or open communication.

Why do patients complain?

- Because they are not given detailed explanations for proposed treatments. Complaints about lack of consent usually only arise after the patient has suffered an adverse event or an unexpected complication. It is best to provide patients with appropriate information and allow patients time to ask questions.
- Because some patients who suffer an adverse event or unanticipated complication are ignored by those responsible for their care and treatment. If detailed explanations about what happened, why it happened and what will be done to help them overcome the problems were provided in a timely manner patients would not complain.
- Because some patients who receive substandard care are not provided with an apology for the inadequacies in the health service.
- Because some health providers do not afford patients dignity and treat them courteously.
- Because some doctors are poor communicators and fail to provide sufficient information and empathy to patients at a time of great vulnerability.

How do complaints help improve medicine?

- They lead to improvements in practice. Clinical decision-making and patient management comprise multiple tasks and complex processes.

There is ample room for error. Complaints can identify particular parts of the process that require review.

- They help to maintain standards. They are one of the ways to identify doctors who are incompetent or unethical. A complaint by a patient can indicate that something may be wrong.
- They provide an alternative to litigation. Most complainants want an explanation about what happened, why it happened and assurances that it won't happen again. If a complaint is taken seriously by the hospital or doctor the complainant is unlikely to seek legal redress.
- They help maintain public trust. Complaints offer patients opportunities to have their concerns about their care examined, but also it acts as a safety valve for other patients if the clinician is practising beyond their limits. Community trust in the profession is maintained because complaints can bring to the attention of the appropriate authorities the wider concern about competence or conduct.
- They encourage self-assessment. Many complaints reflect inadequate communication. Complaints can cause doctors to re-evaluate their communication skills. Irrespective of whether a complaint is justified it provides an opportunity for examining one's communication techniques.
- They remind doctors of their ethical and professional obligations. The stress of receiving a complaint is well documented. Most doctors will receive a complaint against them in their working life; even the most conscientious and skilful clinicians make mistakes. Patient complaints remind doctors of the ethical duties to the patient. Maintaining professional boundaries and putting patient interests ahead of their own interests is paramount. Without complaints the vocational underpinnings of medicine would become weaker. If professionalism weakens so too does the medical profession.

What should you do if you receive a complaint?

You will make mistakes. You are human. Mistakes and complaints are prime learning opportunities and you should view them in this light. Hospitals are complex organisations involving many people in the care of patients, so if you receive a complaint the chances are that other factors will also be involved other than your care and treatment. Poor supervision, tiredness, and inexperience are all factors that contribute to mistakes but these are not the 'fault' of the individual at the point of care resulting in a complaint.

The following are golden rules, which will help you manage complaints and mistakes.

- You should discuss the complaint with your supervisor (clinical tutor, term supervisor, registrar)

- Never lie. If you made a mistake or you don't know what you did it is best to talk it over with your supervisor and he or she will help you understand the issues and help identify remedies. Be frank and honest about what you did and why.
- You should seek out information about how you could avoid repeating the error or conduct that led to the complaint.
- You should speak directly with the patient if appropriate. Apologise if appropriate and let the patient know what you have done to fix the problem.
- The medical records should be appropriately documented.

When a patient suffers a serious adverse event?

- Express sympathy and compassion to the patient or the family. (This will often diffuse a potentially volatile situation.)
- Do not take a defensive position and refrain from castigation or infighting with other members of the healthcare team.
- Do not accept or assign blame or criticise the care or response of other providers.
- Before you make a record in the medical notes discuss the circumstances with an appropriate supervisor.
- Keep the documentation to factual statements of the event and any follow-up required or done as a result of the incident.
- Avoid writing in the record any information unrelated to the care of the patient.

As a junior doctor or medical student you will not be expected to manage the complaint or adverse events alone. Registrars or your supervisors will take the lead in discussions with the patient making the complaint or family members. You can use this opportunity to learn about communications with patients. Observe what works well and what does not.

Associate Professor Merrilyn Walton
Associate Professor of Ethical Practice
Department of Medical Education
Faculty of Medicine
University of Sydney
Sydney, Australia

References

1   Penchansky R, Macnee C. Initiation of medical malpractice suits: a conceptualization and test. *Med Care* 1994; 32:813–31
2   Hingorani M, Wong T, Vafidis G. Patients' and doctors' attitudes to amount of information given after unintended injury during treatment: cross-sectional, questionnaire survey. *BMJ* 1999; 318:640–1

3   Vincent C, Young M, Phillips A. Why do people sue doctors? A study of patients and relatives taking legal action. *Lancet* 1994; 343(8913):1609–13

4   Hickson GB, Clayton EW, Githens PB, Sloan FA. Factors that prompted families to file malpractice claims following perinatal injuries. *JAMA* 1992; 267:1359–63

5   Witman AB, Park DM, Hardin SB. How do patients want physicians to handle mistakes? A survey of internal medicine patients in an academic setting. *Archives of Internal Medicine* 1996; 156(22): 2565–2569

6   Huycke L, Huycke M. Characteristics of potential plaintiffs on malpractice. *Annals of Internal Medicine* 1994; 120(9):792–798

GLOSSARY

A&E	Accident and Emergency
ATN	acute tubular necrosis
AVR	aortic valve replacement
BMA	British Medical Association
CMO	comfort measures only
DNAR orders	Do Not Attempt Resuscitation orders
DoH	Department of Health
DVLA	Driver and Vehicle Licensing Authority
ECG	electrocardiogram
ECT	electro-convulsive therapy
FBC	full blood count
GCS	Glasgow Coma Score
GMC	General Medical Council
HBV	hepatitis B
Hep C+ve	hepatitis C positive
HFEA	Human Fertilisation and Embryology Authority
HIV	human immunodeficiency virus
HRT	hormone replacement therapy
ICD-10	International Classification of Diseases
ICU	intensive care unit
IVF	in-vitro fertilisation
LFT	liver function test
MHAC	Mental Health Act Commission
MHRT	Mental Health Review Tribunal
MMR	measles, mumps and rubella immunisation
MRCP	Member of the Royal College of Physicians

NHS	National Health Service
NR	nearest relative
OCP	oral contraceptive pill
OPD	operating department practitioner
OSCEs	Objective Structured Clinical Examinations
QALYs	quality-adjusted life-years
SSM	Special Study Module
ULTRA	Unrelated Live Transplant Regulatory Authority

APPENDICES

APPENDIX 1: SUGGESTED BOOKS FOR FURTHER READING – AND OUR COMMENTS ON THEM

The Value of Life – An Introduction to Medical Ethics
John Harris
Routledge 1985

Comments: *Easy to read and comprehensive coverage of the issues – philosophical approach and focus.*

Medicine, Patients and the Law
Margaret Brazier
Penguin 1992

Comments: *Good introduction to the legal aspects of medicine in a very readable way. This book provides good analyses of classic cases, but make sure you read more up-to-date sources for the current situation – legal knowledge just like medical knowledge, is constantly developing.*

Principles of Biomedical Ethics
Tom L Beauchamp, James F Childress
Oxford University Press 1994

Comments: *One of the keynote textbooks of medical ethics, focusing on the 'four principles' – covers issues in depth and from a US perspective; will raise antibodies with some ethics teachers if not taken in conjunction with other books and resources.*

Healthy Respect – Ethics in Health Care
Robin Downie and Kenneth Calman
Oxford University Press 1994

Comments: *Very readable, written by a philosopher and the former Chief Medical Officer for England and present Warden of Durham University.*

Wonderwoman and Superman – The Ethics of Human Biotechnology
John Harris
Oxford University Press 1992

Comments: *Looks at the specific area of advancing medical technology and research, and the new ethical issues associated with it.*

Philosophical Medical Ethics
Ranaan Gillon
Wiley 1995

Comments: *Short pithy textbook divided into sections, summarising the ethical issues in medicine.*

Law and Medical Ethics
Mason and McCall Smith
Butterworths 2002 (6th Edition)
Comments: *In-depth textbook focusing on legal issues.*

Medical Ethics Today – its practice and philosophy
British Medical Association
Comments: *A popular and very useful resource book with a wide range of materials relevant to your preparation for essays and examinations.*

Medical Law: Text and Materials
Kennedy and Grubb
Butterworths 2000 (3rd Edition)
Comments: *Very comprehensive textbook with comprehensive and in-depth coverage of all the legal issues.*

Health Care Law
Montgomery
Oxford University Press 2002 (2nd Edition)
Comments: *This is a good primer on health care law.*

Treat Me Right – Essays in Medical Law and Ethics
Ian Kennedy
Oxford University Press, 1996 Edition
Comments: *Challenging, provocative and well worth a read; based on Kennedy's Reith lectures at the BBC in the late 1980s, but still relevant.*

Medical Ethics
Campbell, Charlesworth, Gillett, Jones
Oxford University Press, 1997
Comments: *A good introduction to medical ethics written by well-respected authors based in the UK, Australia and New Zealand.*

Duties of a Doctor
General Medical Council, UK
A series of booklets covering recommendations, requirements and guidance for ethical medical practice in the UK
Comments: *Essential reading.*

APPENDIX 2: USEFUL ADDRESSES

General Medical Council
178 Great Portland Street, London, W1W 5JE, UK
For information on professional ethics email: *standards@gmc-uk.org*
Website: *www.gmc-uk.org*
Tel: 020 7580 7642

British Medical Association
BMA House, Tavistock Square, London, WC1H 9JP, UK
Website: *www.bma.org.uk*
Tel: 020 7387 4499
Email: *info.web@bma.org.uk*

Medical Defence Union
230 Blackfriars Road, London, SE1 8PJ, UK
Website: *www.the-mdu.com*
Tel: 020 7202 1500
Email: *mdu@the-mdu.com*

Medical Protection Society
Granary Wharf House, Leeds LS11 5PY, UK
Website: *www.mps.org.uk*
Tel: 0845 605 4000
Email: *mpsmarketing@mps.org.uk*

Medical and Dental Defence Union of Scotland,
Mackintosh House, 120 Blythswood Street, Glasgow, G2 4EA, UK
Website: *www.mddus.com*
Tel: 0141 221 5858
Email: *info@mddus.com*

Health Service Ombudsman for the UK
Website: *http://www.ombudsman.org.uk/*

Department of Health (UK)
Richmond House, 79 Whitehall, London, SW1A 2NS, UK
Website: *www.doh.gov.uk/index.html*
Tel: 0207 210 4850
Email: *dhmail@doh.gsi.gov.uk*

INDEX

PASTEST BOOKS
FOR
MEDICAL STUDENTS

Essential MCQs for Medical Finals – Second Edition
B Wasan, R Wasan, D Hassanally
- 180 typical finals MCQs with expanded teaching notes
- 3 Practice Exams – 60 MCQs in each
- Tips on exam technique

150 MCQs on Clinical Pharmacology and Therapeutics
D Hassanally & B Wasan
- 3 Practice Exams each containing 50 Multiple Choice Questions
- Detailed answers and expanded teaching notes
- A wide variety of MCQs presented in an easily accessible exam format

Clinical Skills for Medical Students: A Hands-on Guide
Bickle, Hamilton, et al
- Covers system-based chapter i.e. cardiovascular, respiratory with other common examinations
- Useful tips on how to write-up and present a case including case history
- Clear diagrams to explain difficult concepts

Radiology Casebook for Medical Students
R Wasan, A Grundy, R Beese
- Covers X-rays, MR and CT scans
- Read our guidance section to enhance your interpretation skills
- Take the test paper to confirm you are on the right track

EMQs for Medical Students Volumes 1 & 2
A Feather et al
Two volumes of EMQs covering all major themes. Written by doctors at the forefront of medical education with invaluable experience in writing best-sellers for medical students.
- Cover all topics likely to be assessed during medical training
- Over 100 themes contained in each volume
- Essential list of normal values

OSCEs for Medical Undergraduates Volumes 1 & 2
R Visvanathan, A Feather JSP Lumley
Volume 1 covers: Cardiovascular Diseases, Neurology, Psychiatry, Ophthalmology, Otolaryngology, Haematology, respiratory Medicine, Orthopaedics, Trauma, Ethics and Legal Medicine.
Volume 2 covers: Endocrinology, Gastroenterology, Urology, Renal Medicine, Obstetrics, Gynaecology, Rheumatology and Dermatology.
Each book covers:
- History taking, clinical examinations, investigations, practical techniques, making a diagnosis, prescribing treatment and other issues
- Answers and additional information so that you can assess your performance and identify areas needing further attention
- Contain X-rays, scans, haematological and biochemical results and a colour slide section

Surgical Finals: Passing the Clinical
Kuperberg & Lumley
- 90 examples of favourite long and short surgical cases
- Syllabus checklist for structured revision
- 18 detailed examination schemes with action tables
- 36 tables of differential diagnosis
- 134 popular viva questions for self-assessment
- Recommended reading list and revision index.

Medical Finals: Passing the Clinical
Moore & Richardson
- 101 typical long cases, short cases and spot diagnoses
- Syllabus checklist for systematic revision
- Vital tips on preparation and presentation
- Structured examination plans for all cases
- Concise teaching notes highlight areas most relevant to finals
- Revision index for easy access to specific topics

Surgical Finals: Structured Answer and Essay Questions
Visvanathan & Lumley
- Prepare for the written examination with this unique combination of essay questions and the new structured answer questions
- 111 structured answer questions with detailed teaching notes
- 52 typical essay questions with sample essay plans and model essays
- Invaluable revision checklist to help you to trach your progress
- Short textbook reviews enable you to select the best textbooks

Medical Finals: Structured Answer and Essay Questions
Feather, Visvanathan & Lumley
- Prepare for the written examination with this unique combination of essay questions and the new structured answer questions
- 141 structured answer questions with detailed teaching notes
- 73 typical essay questions with sample essay plans and model essays
- Invaluable revision checklist to help you to trach your progress
- Short textbook reviews enable you to select the best textbooks

150 Essential MCQs for Surgical Finals
Hassanally & Singh
- The crucial material for your exam success
- Extended teaching notes, bullet points and mnemonics
- Revision indexes for easy access to specific topics

For priority mail order service, please contact PasTest on 01565 752000, or ORDER ONLINE AT OUR SECURE WEBSITE.

PasTest Ltd, Egerton Court, Parkgate Estate, Knutsford, Cheshire WA16 8DX
Telephone: 01565 752000 Fax: 01565 650264
E-mail: books@pastest.co.uk Website: http//www.pastest.co.uk